PROMOTING INDEPENDENCE FOR OLDER PERSONS WITH DISABILITIES

Assistive Technology Research Series

The Assistive Technology Research Series (ATR) aims to disseminate and archive assistive technology research summaries widely through publishing proceedings, monographs, and edited collective works. The series aspires to become the primary world-wide source of information in assistive technology research, through publishing state-of-the-science material across all continents. ATR defines assistive technology (AT) as any tool, equipment, system, or service designed to help develop, maintain or improve a person with a disability to function in all aspects of his or her life. Assistive technology helps people of all ages who may have a broad range of disabilities or limitations. The ATR series will accept manuscripts and proposals for a wide range of relevant topics.

Volume 18

Recently published in this series

Vol. 19. C. Nugent and J.C. Augusto (Eds.), Smart Homes and Beyond

Vol. 18. W.C. Mann and A. Helal (Eds.), Promoting Independence for Older Persons with Disabilities – Selected Papers from the 2006 International Conference on Aging, Disability and Independence

Vol. 17. H. Mollenkopf, F. Marcellini, I. Ruoppila, Z. Széman and M. Tacken (Eds.), Enhancing Mobility in Later Life – Personal Coping, Environmental Resources and Technical Support. The Out-of-Home Mobility of Older Adults in Urban and Rural Regions of Five European Countries

Vol. 16. A. Pruski and H. Knops (Eds.), Assistive Technology: From Virtuality to Reality – AAATE 2005

Vol. 15. S. Giroux and H. Pigot (Eds.), From Smart Homes to Smart Care – ICOST'2005

Vol. 14. D. Zhang and M. Mokhtari (Eds.), Toward a Human-Friendly Assistive Environment

Vol. 13. H. Mollenkopf, F. Marcellini, I. Ruoppila and M. Tacken (Eds.), Ageing and Outdoor Mobility – A European Study

ISSN 1383-813X

Promoting Independence for Older Persons with Disabilities

Selected Papers from the 2006 International Conference on Aging, Disability and Independence

Edited by

William C. Mann

Rehabilitation Engineering Research Center on Technology for Successful Aging, College of Public Health and Health Professions, University of Florida, Gainesville, FL, USA

and

Abdelsalam Helal

Rehabilitation Engineering Research Center on Technology for Successful Aging, College of Engineering, University of Florida, Gainesville, FL, USA

IOS Press

Amsterdam • Berlin • Oxford • Tokyo • Washington, DC

ISBN 978-1-58603-587-7
Library of Congress Control Number: 2005938587

Second printing, 2007

Publisher
IOS Press
Nieuwe Hemweg 6B
1013 BG Amsterdam
Netherlands
fax: +31 20 687 0019
e-mail: order@iospress.nl

Distributor in the UK and Ireland
Gazelle Books Services Ltd.
White Cross Mills
Hightown
Lancaster LA1 4XS
United Kingdom
fax: +44 1524 63232
e-mail: sales@gazellebooks.co.uk

Distributor in the USA and Canada
IOS Press, Inc.
4502 Rachael Manor Drive
Fairfax, VA 22032
USA
fax: +1 703 323 3668
e-mail: iosbooks@iospress.com

PRINTED IN THE NETHERLANDS

Preface

This book includes 25 full-length papers submitted for the Third International Conference on Aging, Disability, and Independence (ICADI). ICADI was held in St. Petersburg, Florida, USA, from February 1–5, 2006. These papers were submitted under five of the seven ICADI tracks: (1) Smart Homes; (2) Robotics; (3) Telehealth; (4) Home Modifications and Universal Design; and (5) Assistive Devices and Workplace Adaptations. Full-length papers submitted for the Transportation track appear in two special issues of the journal Topics in Geriatrics Rehabilitation published in 2006.

The focus of ICADI, and these papers, is on maintaining independence and active participation in family and community activities. As we age, we face chronic health conditions that have the potential to negatively impact our independence. By using technology (smart homes, robotics, telehealth, other assistive devices), maintaining our mobility, and preventing injuries we can offset much or all of the disabling effects of chronic health conditions.

ICADI brings together a mix of individuals focused on aging, disability and independence, including those involved in research and development, professional practice and services, businesses providing products and services, government and policy planners, and end users and beneficiaries of our research, products, services, and policies. As reflected in this book, ICADI is truly an international conference, with participants from over 45 countries. Assisting us with promotion of this conference, we had close to 100 partner organizations from around the world. In addition, we had 15 sponsors that provided financial support.

This conference, and this book, would not have been possible without the support of the National Institute on Disability and Rehabilitation Research, through the University of Florida Rehabilitation Engineering Research Center on Technology for Successful Aging. The American Occupational Therapy Association served as co-host for ICADI.

The papers in this book provide important content related to aging, disability and independence. They are also a sample of the over 300 ICADI presentations. For those who attended ICADI-2006, this book will provide more in-depth discussion of ICADI presentations. For those who were not able to attend ICADI, this book provides a supplement to the ICADI Conference proceedings, posted at www.icadi.phhp.ufl.edu.

We look forward to seeing all of you at ICADI-2008.

William C. Mann, Abdelsalam Helal
Editors

Contents

Chapter 1

Smart Homes and Robotics

Promoting Independence for Older Persons with Disabilities
W.C. Mann and A. Helal (Eds.)
IOS Press, 2006

Agitation Monitoring of Persons with Dementia Based on Acoustic Sensors, Pressure Sensors and Ultrasound Sensors: A Feasibility Study

Jit BISWAS[a, 1], Maniyeri JAYACHANDRAN[a], Pham Viet THANG[a], Victor Foo Siang FOOK[a], Tay Siew CHOO[a], Qiu QIANG[a], Shiro TAKAHASHI[b], Emily Hao JIANZHONG[b], Chen Jian FENG[c] and Philip Yap Lin KIAT[d]

[a]*Context Aware Systems Department, Institute for Infocomm Research, Singapore*
[b]*Lightwave Department, Institute for Infocomm Research, Singapore*
[c]*Pervasive Signal Processing Department, Institute for Infocomm Research, Singapore*
[d]*Department of Geriatric Medicine, Alexandra Hospital, Singapore*

Abstract: Agitated behavior is common in persons with dementia, and one of the challenges faced by physicians and caregivers is the detailed and continuous monitoring of such persons. With the use of modern sensor and networking technology, and system directed observation, objective outcomes may be expected and with removal of the manpower requirement, evaluation can be continuous and need no longer be confined to clinical settings. In our work we are putting together an observational system composed of multiple sensors of different modalities to collect data from dementia patients in a hospital ward. Through this feasibility study we will gather data to help automate the detection of the onset of agitation in dementia patients. Eventually, with increasing success rates, the sensor based monitoring system and others based on similar concepts, will be effective tools in Smart Home environments for taking detailed observations of the elderly persons' physical activities and behavioral patterns.

Keywords. Agitation monitoring, dementia, sensors

Introduction

Agitated behavior is common in persons with dementia, and one of the challenges faced by physicians and caregivers is the detailed and continuous monitoring of such persons. Due to the detailed nature of the observations that must be taken, time-pressed physicians and over-stressed caregivers are not the ideal people to make detailed records of behavioral patterns of these individuals. Often observations must be made from several angles and along several dimensions such as vocalizations, whole body movements, partial body movements, and repetitive movements. Human observers often tend to miss out on one or more types of behavioral patterns while focusing on a particular pattern of interest, which appears to be the dominant one. It is our belief that with the use of modern sensor and networking technology, and with a combination of multiple algorithmic techniques based on various combinations of sensing modalities, we can be successful in detecting the onset of agitated behavior. Another major benefit is the removal of the manpower requirement. Thus evaluation can be continuous and need no longer be confined to clinical settings. This paper discusses our initial attempt at putting together a system for observing and monitoring a dementia patient in a hospital ward with the purpose of determining the onset and degree of agitation. Note that the results reported in this paper are preliminary, and based on laboratory experimentation, prior to actual deployment of sensors in a hospital ward.

Our work is based on the Scale to Observe Agitation in Persons with Dementia of the Alzheimer Type (SOAPD) [1], developed by Ladislav Volicer, Ann Hurley and Lois Camden, leading world authorities on palliative care for patients with dementia. This tool seeks to objectively classify the degree of agitation experienced by a demented person. Currently, this extremely laborious task is carried out by clinicians who rate the duration of the person's bodily movements and vocalizations every five minutes. For two items (i.e. Repetitive Motions in Place and Outward Motions), intensity of the behavior is also rated. Weights for each behavior, corresponding to the duration and intensity ratings, are given in Table 1. The total score for the observation is then taken to be the summation of the weights for all observed behaviors.

Table 1. Weights for SOAPD Agitation Measurement

Item	Intensity	[1] Duration (d) Short ([2]1) (d < 16s)	Medium ([2]2) (16s ≥ d <2.5m)	Long ([2]3) (2.5m ≥ d <5m)
Total Body Movements (TBM)	N.A	188.9 (= 1*188.9)	377.8 (= 2*188.9)	566.7 (= 3*188.9)
Up and Down Movements (UPM)	N.A	194.2	388.4	582.6
Repetitive Motions in Place (RMP)	Mild ([3]1)	37.3	74.6	111.9
	Moderate([3]2)	98.7	197.4	296.1
	Extreme ([3]3)	191.7	383.4	575.1
Outward Motions (OM)	Mild ([3]1)	36.5	73.0	109.5
	Moderate([3]2)	100.0	200.0	300.0
	Extreme ([3]3)	236.3	472.6	708.9
High Pitched or Loud Words (HLW)	N.A	262.4	524.8	787.2
Repetitive Vocalization (RV)	N.A	179.6	359.1	538.8
Negative Words (NW)	N.A	229.0	458.0	687.0

[1] Duration is specified in seconds (s) and minutes (m).
[2] Value indicates the rating for each duration.
[3] Value indicates the rating for each intensity.

1. Methodology for a partially automated objective assessment

This paper reports our initial work on two of the behavioral features of SOAPD, namely the Total Body Movement (TBM) and Up/Down Movement (UDM) by using multiple modalities of sensors, including ultrasonic sensors and optical fiber grating sensors. In addition we are also investigating the possibility of using microphones for studying the human vocalization related SOAPD indicators, such as High Pitched or Loud Words, Repetitive Vocalization and Negative Words. In the remainder of this section, we discuss the methodology for partially automating TBM and UDM, and the approach for determining vocalization patterns from human voice data captured by microphones.

1.1. Total Body Movement (TBM) and Up/Down Movement (UDM)

The novelty of our approach at detecting TBM and UDM lies in the manner in which sensor data is collected, aggregated, fused and processed in order to reinforce recognition of the features and activities that indicate agitation. For TBM detection, we use ultrasound sensors for accurate recognition and tracking instead of the typical video based solutions which are often considered too intrusive. For UDM detection, we demonstrate the use of two types of sensors working together in concert, namely the Fiber Bragg Grating (FBG) pressure sensor and ultrasound sensor. The fusion of data produced by these two sensing modalities enables more accurate detection.

The FBG pressure sensors are used because fiber optic sensors offer an all-passive dielectric approach that is advantageous in many aspects. These advantages include electrical isolation to prevent shock, elimination of conductive paths in high voltage environments, and immunity to Electromagnetic Interference (EMI). The light-weight, compact and all-solid-state configuration of fiber optic sensors allows them to withstand extreme vibration and even shock. Complementing these attributes are the high sensitivity and large bandwidths of optical fibers, which allows multiplexing of fiber optic sensor arrays. An FBG sensor includes a periodic variation in the refractive index along a specific length of a single-mode optical fiber. When a mechanical pressure/force is applied to an FBG, the internal microstructure of the FBG is disturbed. As a result, there is an expansion or contraction in the grating pitch or the refractive index of the fiber core, which results in the change in Bragg wavelength of the FBG. Hence by detecting the pressure-induced or force-induced wavelength change, we are able to calculate the amount of pressure or force applied on the respective sensor.

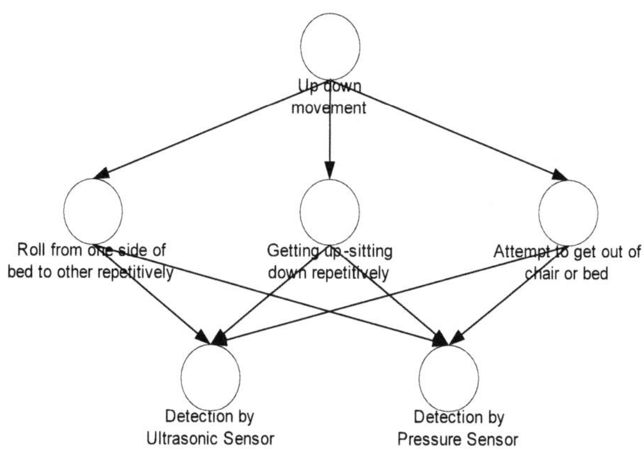

Figure 1. An Example Bayesian Network to deal with Uncertainty and Improve Recognition Rate for Agitation Monitoring

We also study the use of a Bayesian network shown in Figure 1, to perform data fusion and inference to improve the recognition rate and to deal with uncertainty. Due to the unpredictable behavior patterns of patients and uncontrollable sensor reading errors, an inference engine, such as a Bayesian network, is necessary for any reliable report on agitation behavior detection given evidence from sensors. In our approach, we initially obtain a set of sample data from experiments, and use this set of sample data to train the Bayesian networks. In the real-life environment, such trained Bayesian networks are used to fuse the readings from multiple modalities of sensors. Some experimental results are included in a later section to prove the feasibility of agitation monitoring using ultrasound and FBG pressure sensors.

1.2. High Pitched or Loud Words, Repetitive Vocalization and Negative Words

The signal of the patient's vocalization is relatively easy to obtain. Two condenser microphones are used in the testing environment to capture all the sounds during the diagnostic observation periods. Our preliminary experiments and analysis show that based on the existing technologies it would be reasonably straightforward to measure "high pitched" or "loud words" at a rather acceptable accuracy. On the other hand, some difficulties are also identified. For example, it would not be that straightforward to mark "repetitive vocalizations." Elaborated vocal models should be designed before the "repetition" could be searched. As for the "negative words," their detection and identification is even more challenging, since they may relate to notions of human emotion classification, speech/language recognition and even the high level speech understanding. Nevertheless, it has been illustrated that in many cases the investigator may not necessarily understand what the patient is saying when marking the "negative words" score.

2. Implementations & Results:

2.1. Hardware Setup

The prototype system consists of 10 ultrasound sensor nodes as shown in Figure 2, used to detect total body movement, and 1 ultrasound sensor node and a seat pressure sensor pad using an array of FBG sensors to detect disturbed up down movement as shown in Figure 3. The ultrasound sensors are mounted at the level of the ceiling, as illustrated in the mock-up frame depicted in Figures 2 and 3.

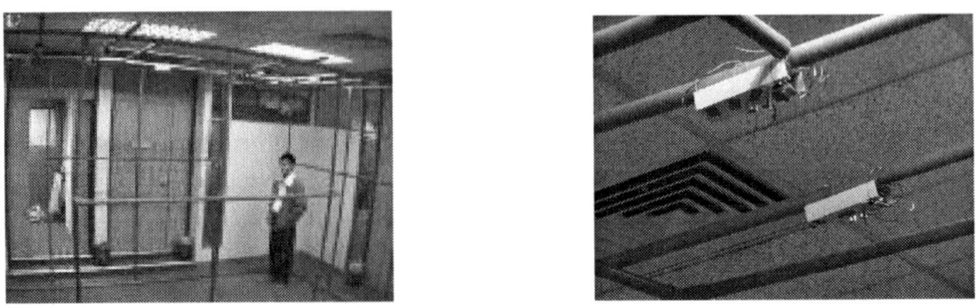

Figure 2. Setup for Total Body Movement (TBM) Detection

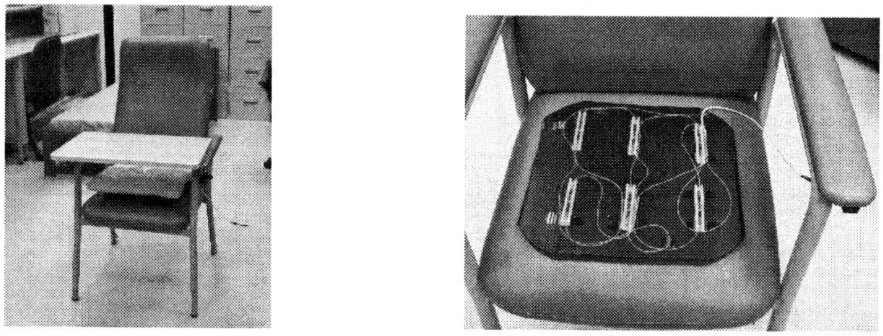

Figure 3. Setup for Up Down Movement (UDM) Detection

Each of the ultrasound sensors is equipped with a Micaz mote developed by Crossbow [2]. The mote has an inbuilt ATMEL MEGA128L processor and a CC1000 radio component with a transmission range of 100 feet. Each mote has a 51 pin connector which includes 8 power pins and a few general purpose I/O pins through which the ultrasound sensors can be interfaced to the processor board. The mapping of the registers of the processor to the interface pins is given in the hardware manual of ATMEL128, and the driver program for control of the sensor is written in assembly language. The assembly instructions are executed using NESC code, a simple programming language developed in the University of California at Berkeley and used widely in wireless sensors. For choice of ultrasound sensor, we use SRF04 ultrasound sensor from Devantech Ltd. [3] for sensing the range of the patient as shown in Figure 4. The SRF04 ultrasound sensor offers precise ranging information from roughly 3 cm to 3 meters which suits our needs and is low cost. The ultrasound sensor is connected to the processor board which indicates the 4 pins of the sensor, i.e. Voltage source (Vcc), Echo Line, Trigger line and Ground, and the mapping of pins from ultrasonic sensor to the processor is shown in Figure 4.

Processor – Pin# , Port	Ultrasonic sensor
Power 0 – Pin 29 , C0	Voltage Source (Pin 0)
General I/O – Pin 3 , E7	Trigger Line (Pin 3)
General I/O – Pin 6, E4	Echo Line (Pin 2)
Ground – Pin 0	Ground (Pin 4)

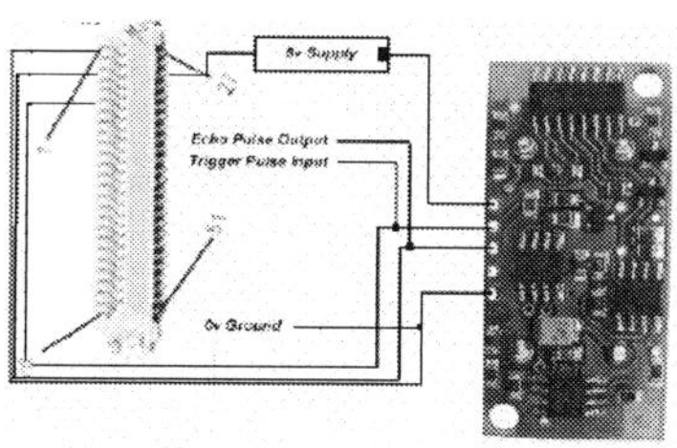

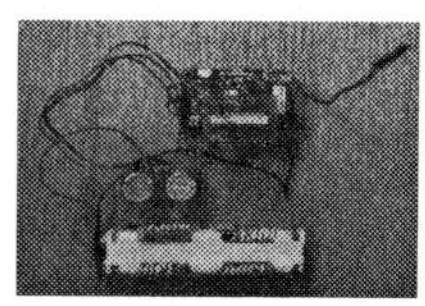

Figure 4. Ultrasonic Sensor integrated to Mote Platform

2.2. Optical Fiber based Pressure Sensors

The seat pressure sensor pad consists of six FBG sensor points along a single fiber to form a seat pressure sensor pad as shown in Figure 5(a) and 5(b). Each FBG is 5mm long, embedded at the center of some carbon fiber reinforced composite material with a lamination sequence of 0/0/0/FBG/0 and then made into a four-point bending structure.

Calibration on Bragg wavelength of FBG versus vertically applied force is carried out with very good linearity as shown in Figure 6.

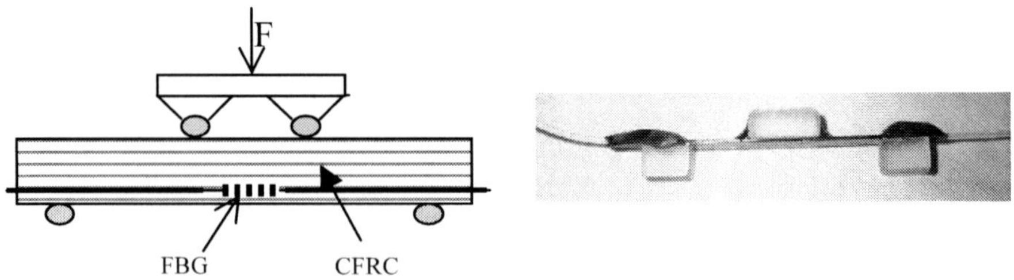

(a) Structure b) Real picture

Figure 5 Structure of each FBG sensor (the 5mm long FBG is embedded at the center of some carbon fiber reinforced composite (CFRC) material with a lamination sequence of 0/0/0/FBG/0 and then made into a four-point bending structure)

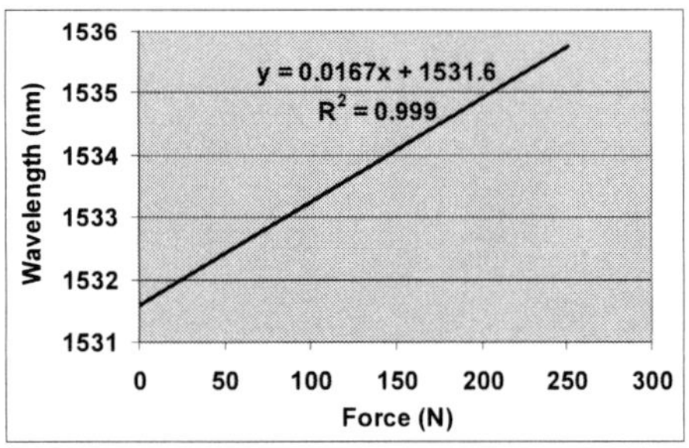

Figure 6. Calibration results between Bragg wavelength of FBG and vertically applied force

2.3. Software Infrastructure

Figure 7 shows the software infrastructure of our prototype system. It consists of the sensor nodes, sensor node server, and central server with Bayesian inference engine and a server for the web-browser based user interface.

Sensor nodes may be of various modalities. For the purpose of this paper, the sensor nodes are ultrasound sensors or FBG pressure sensors. Sensor node servers are mote base station for ultrasound sensors or the FBG interrogation unit for the FBG pressure sensor. In order to equip the sensors for deployment in a service oriented architecture, they are Universal Plug and Play (UPnP) enabled, since UPnP offers a standard-based, dynamic and flexible architecture for devices of widely differing capabilities. This is important as our system would predictably involve the use of a wide range of sensors. As it is designed to support zero-configuration and automatic discovery of devices, the ability to replace these sensors or reconfigure them with minimal effort would give great potential for our system in practical use. The sensor node server is responsible for raw data processing in the test-bed. It implements data fusion, association and activity tracking algorithms, and executes them whenever it receives raw data from the sensor nodes, and inserts the data with or without fusion into the local database. To support real time application, we decompose the sensor data as three levels consisting of raw, aggregated and summarized levels. Raw level data are data with pre-processing but without analysis. Aggregated level data are data/information for multi-sensors of the same modality with pre-processing and analysis, i.e., after feature extraction and classification.

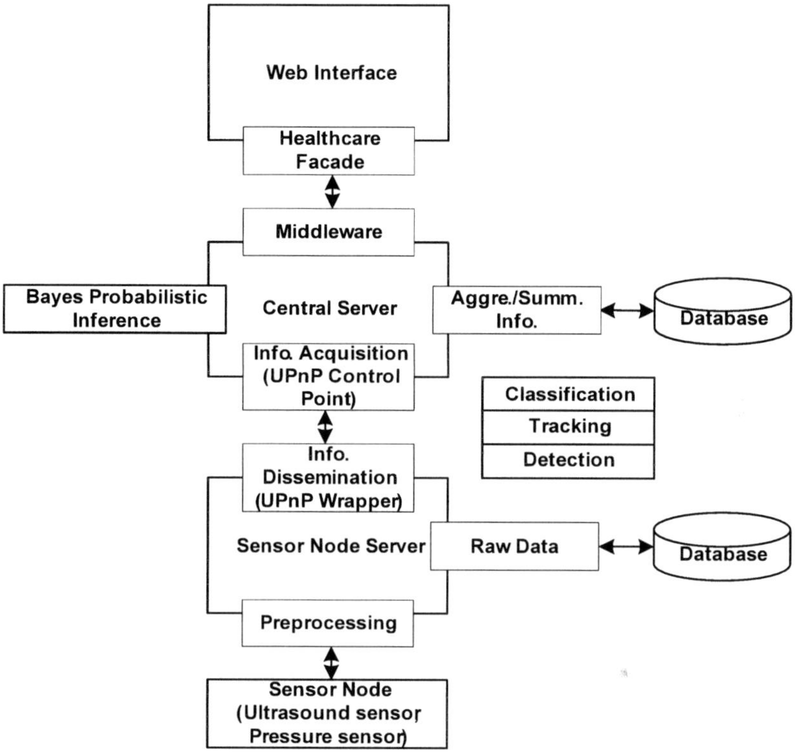

Figure 7. Software Infrastructure

Likewise, summarized level data are data/information for sensors with different sensor modality with pre-processing and analysis. The raw data is kept in the local database and only summarized level and aggregated level information are allowed to be sent to the central server from the node server. This promotes scalability by restricting the flow of high volume data through wireless networks that are close to the environment while capturing important features of the data and capturing them in the central database. The information being sent to the central server is indexed by time. The value of time is obtained from a server using the Network Time Protocol (NTP) protocol. The UPnP control point in the central server coordinates the discovery of information and subscription of events between the central server and the node server. There is also a Bayesian engine in the server for performing information fusion between sensors of different modalities, and a web server for building standard web based user interface for visualization.

3. Experiment

3.1. Total Body Movement - Sensor Interference and Scheduling

We started our experiments on ultrasound sensors for disturbed total body movement by deploying them at ceiling level, and a person working back and forth according to the typical pattern of pacing by dementia patient when they are agitated. When we conducted our experiments, we found that there are a lot of wrong range measurements when the ultrasound sensors are located near each other. We found that this is due to inter-sensor interference when the wave emitted by one ultrasound sensor is received by another ultrasound sensor and wrongly considered by the receiving sensor as its own echo wave. We found that the two main reasons which cause the interference are distance between sensors and sampling rate. Our experiment shows that, if the height of sensor is around 2.5m, the optimal distance between sensors is 0.7m and the sampling rate is 2 samples per second.

To overcome this problem, we have implemented a mechanism to schedule the sensors wisely, meaning that sensors are turned on and off at the right time, reducing as much as possible, the interference presented to other sensors. We call it *time division scheduling.*

The basic idea of time division scheduling is to make sure there is one and only one sensor operating at any given time. The sensors work in a round-robin manner. Each sends out its signal, and then comes to idle state, waiting for all the others to send their signals and then activates sending its signal, and returns to idle state again. At the beginning, when we turn on all the sensors, each sensor has different delay time before sending its signal, but then all the sensors are programmed with the same "sleep interval." The computation of how long each sensor should go to sleep and how long is the delay for each sensor at the beginning depends on the number of sensors in the sensor network and the sampling rate we would like to have from each individual sensor.

3.2. Up Down Movement – Multiple Sensor Modality Data Fusion

We also carried out a set of experiments on the chair for disturbed up down movement, with a person showing typical movement of dementia patient seated in a locked chair.

In addition to the data on agitation detection reported by each modality of sensors, a series of time-stamped manual observations are also required for the training set. During the training data collection phase, whenever agitation behavior of patients is observed, some simple input mechanisms, e.g., through pressing anywhere on the keyboard, are used to notify the system the current timestamp. The training data are further processed based on the criteria shown in Table 1, to obtain a combined agitation record from both manual observations and sensor detections. For example, for the short duration agitation detection, the time domain is uniformly divided into 16-second slices and a binary value is assigned to each time slice for both manual observation and detection of sensors from each modality, with '1' indicating the presence of agitation presence and '0' for no agitation observed. Such processed binary values are used to compute the Conditional Probability Table (CPT) for constructing a Bayesian network.

4. Results:

4.1. Total Body Movement

With the ceiling deployment as above, we expect to be able to able to monitor the total body movement as well as up-down movement in real-life settings in the hospital ward. Since the data we have from ultrasonic sensor is the distance from sensor to the nearest object, obviously the person should be under the sensor which gives us the smallest reading. This simple rule is also the basic of our data fusion algorithm. Whenever we have data sent from one of the ultrasound sensors, we create a matrix which represents the current reading value of all these sensors. In our deployment, the size of this matrix is 2x5. Scanning this matrix, and finding the minimum element, we may assume the corresponding sensor would be the location of the person in the room. Figure 8 shows the reading from 10 sensors when the person is moving. At any given time, the shortest bar represents the position of the person in the room. The trajectory then has the format like an array of boxes. We also record the time when the person moves from one sensor to another, so we know duration of staying under each sensor up to the nearest millisecond. We repeated our experiment several times by letting a person walking under the sensors. Our system recorded correctly, the position of the person in the room 90% of the time.

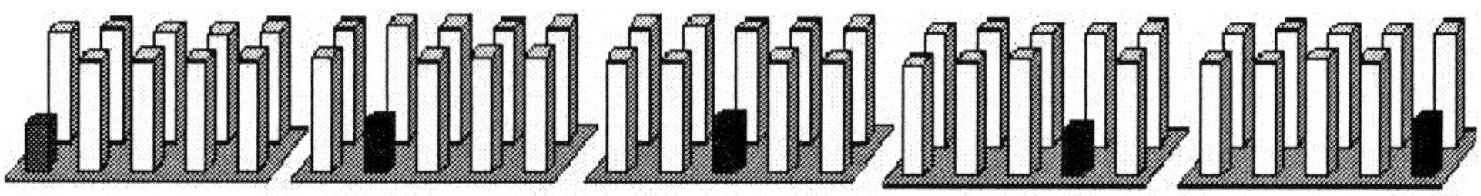

Figure 8. Continuous reading from 10 sensors.
The shortest bar (dark colored) represents the position of the person in the room.

4.2. Up/Down Movement

If a person sitting in a chair under one sensor, we believe that our ceiling deployment can detect the up and down behavior of the person. Figure 9 shows the data from one sensor when a person repeats the up and down movement.

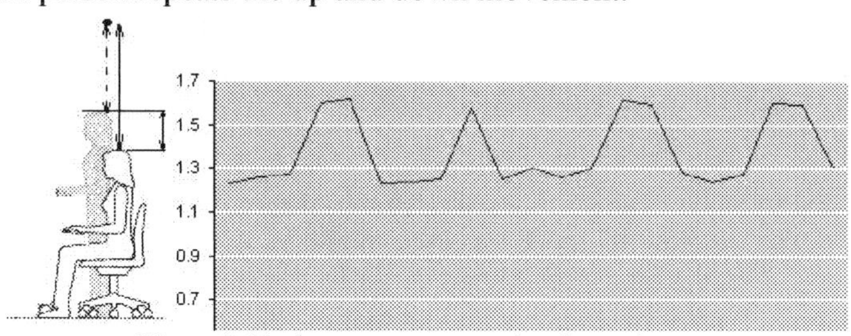

Figure 9. Up down movement under ultrasonic sensor

Several humps in the data show the times at which the person is moving towards standing up position. Our data fusion for up and down behavior uses the current reading from the sensor and maintains a window frame of its past reading. By observing the relation between current reading value and the previous ones, we know whether the person changes his/her posture between sitting and standing. The pseudo-code of our algorithm is shown below. We define two states: sitting - standing and maintain a window of past value of size L. We also need a threshold between sitting and standing. We calculate the sum S of all the differences between the current value and each value in the window.

```
if (currState==STANDING)
        if (sum(S) > threshold)
        currState=SITTING;
else
        if (sum(S) < - threshold)
                currState=STANDING;
```

The parameters *size of window* L, and *threshold* need to be tuned depends on the different application. We do several experiment of up and down detection. The result shows that for normal person fully standing, window size may be L=3 and threshold=15cm, and we can detect the up down movement correctly 90% of the time. But the dementia patient, who is seated in a locked chair is unable to do move to the fully standing position, but only able to do a semi-standing position. In this case, the two parameters should be L=4 and threshold=8cm. In this case our algorithm is able to recognize up and down movement correctly between 50% and 70% of the time. Note that these results are for ultrasound sensors only, and do not assume any data fusion with other modalities.

4.3. Pressure Sensor.

The pressure sensor gives a continuous value of amplitude phase shift. In this case, there are 6 FBG sensor points created along one single fiber. We threshold the values from each of these sensor points into 4 levels at a sampling rate of 25 Hz, and at each point in time, we obtain 6 values coming from the 6 pressure sensor points. We obtain the feature vector x(t) and data set D over a period of time (row vector of dataset D is called time vector while the column vector is defined a feature vector).

D=[x1(t1)…x1(tn)

……………..

xd(t1)…x6(tn)]

4.4. Pressure Sensor Detection Algorithm.

In our first prototype we used simple algorithm based on averaging of the matrix across rows and columns. A threshold value was chosen based on experimental observation and when the average pressure was below this threshold, the patient was assumed to be UP from his seat and when the average was above this threshold, the patient was assumed to be in sitting or DOWN position.

A state machine was implemented to start monitoring when the patient sits on the chair and to stop monitoring when he/she leaves the chair for long duration. When the first UP-DOWN movement was detected, we continued to monitor for another 16 seconds for the number of UP-DOWN movements. The level of agitation was assumed to be LOW when the number of UP-DOWN movements within this period was more

than a threshold, decided based on experimental observation. We will be extending this algorithm in future
to cover cases of HIGH agitation.

4.5. Bayesian Information Fusion

In UDM detection, owing to the mutually supplementary functions of ultrasound and FBG pressure sensors in capturing information, the following possible behavior patterns are observed during experiments:

1. While agitated, patients may only trigger ultrasonic sensors but not pressure sensors by avoiding constantly touching the surface where the pressure sensors are deployed.
2. While agitated, patients may only trigger pressure sensors but not ultrasonic sensors by moving body with high intensity but low amplitude.
3. While not agitated, patients may still trigger pressure sensors but not ultrasonic sensors by adjusting body position normally but frequently.

The fused results from ultrasound and FBG sensors given by a Bayesian network provide us a much high agitation recognition rate than that given by the individual modalities, as shown in Table 2.

Table 2. Experiment Results on Agitation Recognition Rate Improvement with Multi-Modalities Sensor Fusion through Bayesian Inference

Sensor Modality	Agitation Recognition Rate
Ultrasonic sensor alone	59 %
FBG pressure sensor alone	75 %
Both Ultrasonic and FBG Pressure Sensor with Bayesian Inference	94 %

Preliminary results in the laboratory are quite encouraging and indicate a very significant detection rate of TBM even without multi-modal information fusion. For UDM the recognition rates through single modality are not very good because of the fine granularity of the motion. However, with multi-modal information fusion between the ultrasonic and pressure sensing modalities, we expect that even in the real-life setting in the hospital ward, the recognition rates will be significantly improved, as illustrated in our preliminary experimental results from our laboratory. These results are being validated in the hospital environment in a data collection exercise scheduled to end in December 2005.

5. Conclusions

The monitoring of elderly people is going to be increasingly important in the coming years, as a means of facilitating their independent living in their homes. For persons with dementia it is important for both the patient (for early detection of stress and agitation), and the care-giver (for relief from continuous detailed monitoring tasks), that automated, non-obtrusive means of monitoring be developed. Our research is a first step in this direction. In concurrent work we are looking at several other modalities including video and acoustic, and classifying other patterns of behavior. It is expected that with increasing success rates of detection, these technologies can be deployed in the patients' homes.

References

[1] Ann C. Hurley, et al., "Measurement of Observed Agitation in Patients with Dementia of the Alzheimer's Type," Journal of Mental Health and Aging, 1999.
[2] Crossbow Technology, http://www.xbow.com.
[3] Devantech Ltd. (Robot Electronics), http://www.robot-electronics.co.uk.

Promoting Independence for Older Persons with Disabilities
W.C. Mann and A. Helal (Eds.)
IOS Press, 2006

Developing a Well-Being Monitoring System – Modeling & Data Analysis Techniques

Steve BROWN[a,1], Basim MAJEED[a], Nicholas CLARKE[b], Beum-Seuk LEE[b]
[a]*Research & Venturing, British Telecom PLC, Adastral Park, Ipswich IP5 3RE, UK.*
[b]*Dept. of Engineering Mathematics, University of Bristol, Bristol BS8 1TR, UK.*

Abstract. This paper describes how the DTI funded 'Care in the Community Centre' led by British Telecom PLC (UK), has developed a concept model to represent an individual's well-being. The paper goes on to provide an in-depth explanation of the data analysis techniques used to monitor changes in well-being. By combining related sensor events (sensors in the activity based sensor groups), the activity of the client can be inferred. This not only provides an overall assessment and better representation of the data but also highlights significant (i.e. noteworthy) events. The aim to provide caregivers with a tool that enables them to make more appropriate and timely decisions regarding the well-being of their clients. The social interaction of the client with visitors is used as an example activity and is explained in detail to show the capabilities of the system. The data pre-processing and analysis techniques used are heavily reliant on fuzzy sets and fuzzy reasoning techniques in order to deal with the vagueness and incompleteness of the data.

Keywords. Telecare, well-being, monitoring system, activities of daily living

Introduction

Telecare can be described as the use of information and communication technology (ICT) to support independent living for older, frail and disabled people. Telecare is not a new concept; in fact telecare solutions have been available for several years from suppliers in Europe and the US, and many telecare trials are in operation today [1]. Many of these existing telecare solutions have been used successfully and have proven to be cost effective in addition to saving lives. But the fundamental aim of these existing solutions is to alert a carer to an immediate problem where, for example, a person has become incapacitated, or is in immediate danger within their own home. We refer to these existing systems as 1st and 2nd generation telecare systems. The difference between 1st and 2nd generation telecare is the way in which an alert is generated: 1st generation telecare relies upon the person themselves activating the alert through the use of a pull cord attached to the ceiling, or a pendent worn around the neck and connected wirelessly to a base station receiver within the home. However, in cases where the person is unable to raise the alert, or may feel they do not want to disturb a carer, then the system becomes ineffective. To remedy this some telecare solutions have progressed to monitoring particular activities or inactivity within the home through the use of ambient sensors. These systems incorporate a degree of intelligence allowing an alert to be raised automatically. These intelligent systems are known as 2nd generation telecare systems.

Advances in sensor design and the continuing reduction in the cost of processing data mean that it is now becoming practical to develop a new generation of telecare capable of monitoring the general well-being of an individual. We call this 3rd generation telecare and its aim is to *prevent* incidents from occurring within the home rather than just *responding* to them. BT's Care in the Community Centre [2] is developing such a system.

1. A Working Model for Well-Being

There is an underlying idea that well-being is in some way about the 'goodness' in someone's life, but beyond this there appears to be no straightforward or agreed definition. In order to build a system capable of monitoring changes in well-being, it is first necessary to develop an understanding of what constitutes well-being for frail older people. Essentially a working definition, framework or model is required. The model of well-being used within the Care in the Community Centre is based upon a definition for well-being as used by the World Health Organization [3]. This definition suggests that well-being consists of three separate but interrelated components: mental well-being, social well-being and physical well-being. We believe each of these components, and hence our overall or general well-being, is determined by our experiences of everyday life, and our experiences are determined by the activities we perform, or in some cases fail to perform. In addition to this our experiences of performing or not performing activities are affected by personal and context factors, which also affect the type of activities we perform.

Current methods used by carers for determining changes in an individual's well-being are based upon observing the individual and asking them relevant questions about their everyday lives. However, many older individuals are fiercely independent and may not always be willing to provide honest answers if they believe this might lead to a loss of independence or might create extra burden for a carer. Observing an individual in this way provides only snap-shots of their well-being, the frequency of which will be dependent upon the resources of the carer. For this reason, ambient sensors can be deployed to monitor specific activities within the home, to provide more detailed information about the individual to the appropriate carer. The carer could use this information in conjunction with their observations to create a more detailed, accurate and constant understanding of changes to the well-being of that individual.

A number of activities have been identified for monitoring through the use of ambient sensors. These activities can be grouped into three categories:

- Social interaction: meeting people inside and outside of the home.
- Personal goals: activities which give meaning and interest in life such as hobbies, caring for others and one's self.
- ADL's (Activities of Daily Living): basic but important activities such as cooking, washing, cleaning etc.

We have identified many activities within each of these categories which could be monitored, and there are probably many more. However, modeling how an individual might perform each of these activities in order to identify changes that might affect well-being is a very complex task that is beyond the resources available to this project. For this reason the initial focus was on the frail elderly target group, with a restricted number of activities, these are:

- Leaving and returning home
- Receiving visitors
- Preparing food and eating
- Sleeping patterns
- Personal appearance
- Leisure activities

The following sections will present the data analysis methodology used to convert the raw sensor data to the kind of information that provides the carer with the status of each of these activities.

2. Analysis Techniques

2.1. Abstract Activities of Daily Living

The intended end result of this project is a user interface to assist the care professionals in making informed decisions about the well-being status of the monitored person. In the context of well-being monitoring, three aspects are important: long-term trends, significant patterns, and associations among patterns. The long-term trend analysis is needed to answer the questions related to changes over a significant time period. For example the carer might want to find out whether the duration of the main sleep-period is increasing or decreasing, or whether the client is changing the location of the main sleep period (e.g. from the bedroom to the living room). The pattern discovery finds the events that occur frequently or regularly (e.g., on most Sundays there might be evidence of visitors and of a substantial meal being prepared). The association analysis discovers the patterns that occur together and strength of association between them (e.g., the client might take a bath before going out on Monday mornings). Finally, any activity changes related to the well-being status are reported to the caregiver on demand. All the substantial or gradual changes in daily activities are reported to the client's care-giver with the detailed analysis conveyed in a fashion allowing a non-expert in data analysis to easily understand the results.

To carry out intelligent analyses, the sensors are grouped together according to the domain knowledge and specific activities of interest [4]. Each sensor may belong to more than one sensor group, thus allowing the fusion of the large amount of raw sensor data streams into structures that represent higher level (Abstract) activities. By maintaining these groups, analyses using individual or environment specific information focus only on the relevant sensors. An overview of the proposed analysis is shown in Figure 1.

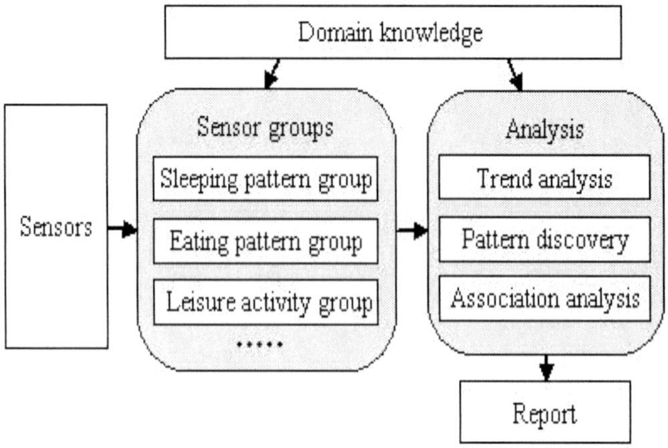

Figure 1. An overview of the analysis process for well-being monitoring.

2.2. B. Sensor Choice and Data Pre-Processing

The sensors installed at the client's house can be classified into two types: location sensor type and activity sensor type. The location sensor type is usually a passive infrared (PIR) sensor that is used to detect the location of the client and the level of movement in that location. The second type of sensor provides information on the specific interaction that the client performs (or the lack of interactions) with appliances such as the fridge, toilet flush, bed occupancy and the water supply. The location of the client is the most crucial information in well-being analysis as activities are strongly related to location. It is necessary to provide the location information with a high degree of confidence in order to make correct inferences about the abstract activities. The problem with sensor choice, in particular those with specialized function, however is the fact that clients can be sensitive to having them installed in their home. For example, the client may not be comfortable with anything other than a PIR sensor in the bathroom for reasons of privacy. In this case, activities in the bathroom must be inferred by looking at how much time the person spends in the room and the time of day it is occupied. On the other hand, using only a PIR sensor in the kitchen would not be sufficient to infer what the client is doing in that location confidently. Several activities (eating, preparing food, merely passing through the kitchen to get to another room, getting food from the fridge, etc.) may occur with similar duration at any time of day, rendering them indistinguishable.

Having an insufficient number of sensors isn't the only problem that can hinder the analysis process in drawing confident conclusions. There are situations where a sensor is not triggered as expected (e.g., a PIR sensor is blocked by a door) or two PIR sensors in the current room and in a nearby room are triggered at the same time. The latter case may not be easily distinguished from the case when there is a visitor or a second occupant. (The current project is initially restricted to single-occupancy cases.)

The above mentioned factors indicate strongly that in addition to ensuring the proper installation and maintenance of the sensors and the network, the information of the layout of the client's house and the location choice of each sensor are extremely important issues in guaranteeing a robust system. Locating the sensors in the home of the client should not be carried out in an ad hoc manner, and a proper study of the layout of the home and the way in which PIR sensors relate/interfere with each other are necessary before installation. With a thorough design of sensor location in conjunction with an understanding of the type of activities the client is engaged in, rules for data pre-processing and correction of erroneous readings can be implemented. The same information is also used to overcome environment dependencies in analysis caused by clients having unique house layouts.

Other than the location of each sensor, the ranges for the expected values and significant values are used to filter out erroneous or insignificant events. For example, the person is not normally expected to spend over 12 hours in the kitchen, whilst bed occupancy duration of less than one minute may not be of interest or significance.

Sensor data, whether raw or pre-processed, are unlikely to be meaningful to the end user, who will be more likely to think in terms of possible problems at a higher level (i.e. Abstract Activities). Therefore the analysis needs to follow a qualitative reporting approach that is easy to understand by the users. In addition, reporting the state of the client's well-being also requires a justification on how and why the system has reached such a particular conclusion. A rule-based fuzzy logic [5] system turns out to be a good candidate for this purpose as it not only allows the rules to be specified in a controlled manner, but also it can keep track of the rules that have been fired to obtain a certain result.

2.3. Fuzzification of Input Data

A daily activity can occur at an arbitrary time of day and usually with a variety of durations. There are several important factors regarding sensor events that are significant with regards to the person's well-being. The time of day when the event occurs, the duration of the event, the frequency of the event, and the day of week when the event occurs are just some examples of these factors. For illustrative purposes, only the first two factors and the sensor name are considered in this paper.

The quantitative values, namely the time the sensor is triggered (StartTime) and the duration the sensor has been active since its first activation (Duration), are discredited using fuzzy membership functions [6]. The fuzzy membership functions for StartTime segment the whole day into 12 overlapping groups (EarlyDawn, Dawn, LateDawn, EarlyMorning, Morning, LateMorning, EarlyAfternoon, Afternoon, LateAfternoon, EarlyEvening, Evening, and LateEvening). Its partial fuzzy membership graph is shown in Figure 2.

Unlike the fuzzy membership functions for the Start Time, constructing the fuzzy memberships for Duration is rather complex. Each sensor has to have its own Duration membership functions because the duration ranges significantly vary depending on the sensors. To construct these fuzzy membership functions statistical measures such as average and semi-quartile range values were used. Figure 3 shows the fuzzy membership function for the Kitchen Duration variable.

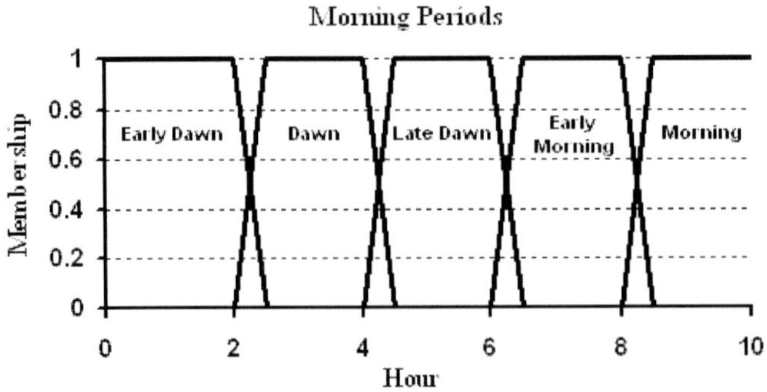

Figure 2. Fuzzy membership function for the Start Time variable.

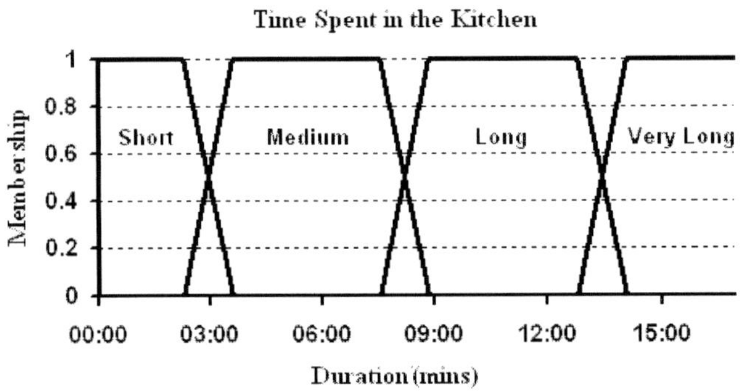

Figure 3. Fuzzy membership function for kitchen activity.

3. Visitor Interaction Activity

In the previous sections, a well-being model was identified, and sensor data was pre-processed. The next stage is to see how an abstract activity is deduced and how it is presented to the user. As an example, the visitor interaction activity will be discussed. This was a particularly interesting activity because it was not straightforward to identify whether there are other persons in the home apart from the occupant, or whether, in the case when there is only one person in the home, the person is the client. It was a decision made at the beginning of the project not to use any identification tags or video imaging equipment. This decision was a result of a study which concluded that most potential clients will not accept sensors that might be perceived as intruding on their privacy. In the following discussion, the pre-processing specifically needed for this activity is presented; this is followed by how fuzzy reasoning is applied to determine likely visitor periods and the confidence with which these are determined.

3.1. Pre-processing with Fuzzy Membership Functions

The data in Figure 4 shows triggers from the motion sensors detected (white) during a one-hour period in the home of a single occupant. The data segment has been split into three regions (A, B, C) according to the entrance events observed, such that each region denotes a time during which the number of persons in the home should remain constant.

By comparing the behaviors exhibited in regions neighboring an entrance event, it is possible to determine those likely to correspond with persons arriving, leaving, or simply interacting with someone on the doorstep.

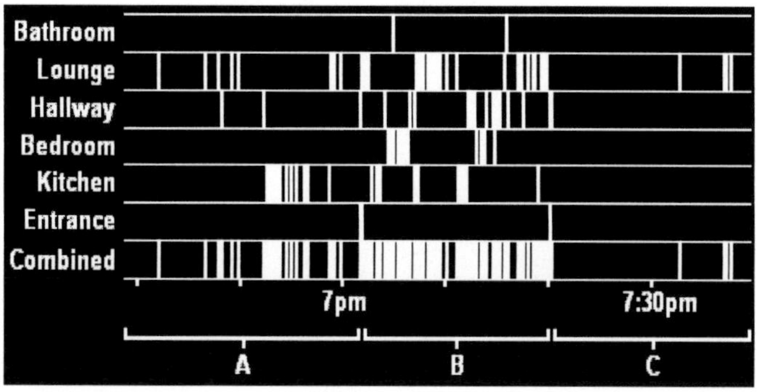

Figure 4. An example of motion sensor data.

Several characteristics of neighboring regions may be compared, the choice of which being constrained by the type of data available. From the data gathered so far in the trials, the following fuzzy-based comparisons were made (Note that Figure 4 serves as an example case, and that regions A and C continue beyond the boundaries of the graphic).

1. *Activity Level* is defined as the proportion of time in which movements or object use was detected, so visually this is the average density of the white areas in the combined row for regions in Fig 4. The assumption made is that as more people enter the home, so on average the number of activities detected will rise. The difference in levels between the regions is converted to a fuzzy value according to the membership function of Fig 5. Similarly the other measures are also converted to suitable fuzzy descriptions, serving as the inputs for rules to classify the door events.

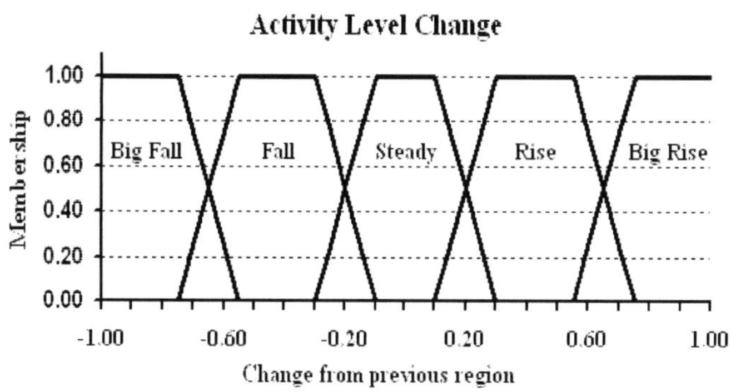

Figure 5. Fuzzy sets denoting change in activity levels.

2. *Changing Rooms Level* is a measure of how often the room in which activities are currently detected changes. It is assumed that as visitors enter the home, some activities will take place simultaneously in different rooms, causing the data to apparently show very frequent changes. The value returned is the mean of the rate of apparent room changes, and the proportion of room changes deemed impossible for one person to make, as is the case for non-adjacent rooms.
3. *Delay Time* is a measure of how long it takes before the activity level shows signs of the change recorded. This is obtained by use of a sliding window, and the delay is the time taken before the activity level within the window is closer to the activity level for the second region than the first. In Figure 6, the very first window has an activity level closer to that of region B than A; hence the delay time in this case is zero, an instantaneous change. Short delays such as this are consistent with changes to the number of persons in the home, while long delays are more consistent with a coincidental later change in behavior, such as a person becoming more active to cook dinner.

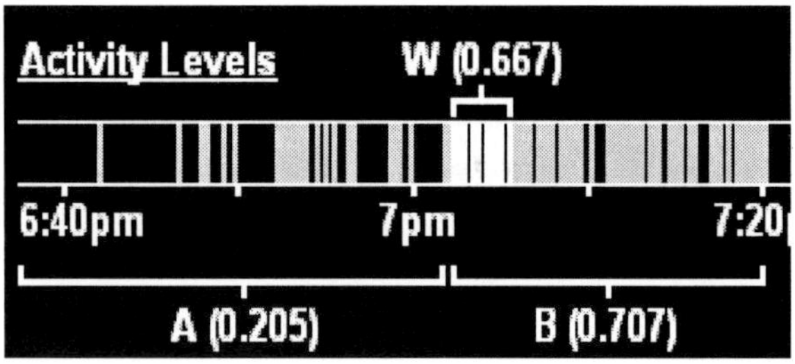

Figure 6. Activity levels for regions A, B, and a sliding window W.

4. *Hallway Time* either side of a door event adds more clues, such as whether or not a person has been let in, seen out, or is taking off and unpacking some items after coming inside. Unfortunately the data used to calculate this period is difficult to accurately assess, as the data may show a change in room because of a single person leaving the hall, or a second person moving in another room.
5. *Door Open Time* is the time during which the door was open. Longer times imply a higher likelihood of visitors remaining outside if there is no evidence of others entering the home; otherwise, a long time is consistent with guests bringing items inside.

Once the data has been converted into fuzzy descriptions, rules can be applied to describe the likelihood that visitors did indeed arrive and leave during those door events.

4. The User Interface (GUI) Components

Users interact with the system using a number of GUI components such as the sensor management component and the parameter setting component. The component of main interest however, is the data display and analysis component which displays the analysis results to the caregiver. The GUI is split into two main components, namely the calendar view and the analysis reporting views. These views are discussed below together with some of the data analysis aspects behind them.

4.1. A. The Calendar View

The calendar view is shown in Figure 7 in grayscale. The original view uses a coloring scheme to convey information to the user. This view allows the user to select individual days for detailed examination, and highlights days where unusual activity has taken place. The colored controls on the calendars indicate the normality of the daily patterns. The dates in any of yellow, blue, or green colors are likely to contain unusual events in comparison to the learned normal behavior according to the following scheme:

- Yellow indicates the amount of normally occurring events that are missing.
- Blue represents the amount of unusual extra events observed.
- Green illustrates a combination of both missing and extra events.
- Pale Red means the day is ignored in the analysis process, usually because the day doesn't have enough data due to sensor or communication failure.

The intensity of color (apart from red) indicates the degree of abnormality, so a brighter yellow indicates a greater number of missing events for example. The normal behavior is learned from the history of the data using a combination of fuzzy logic, statistics and association rule mining.

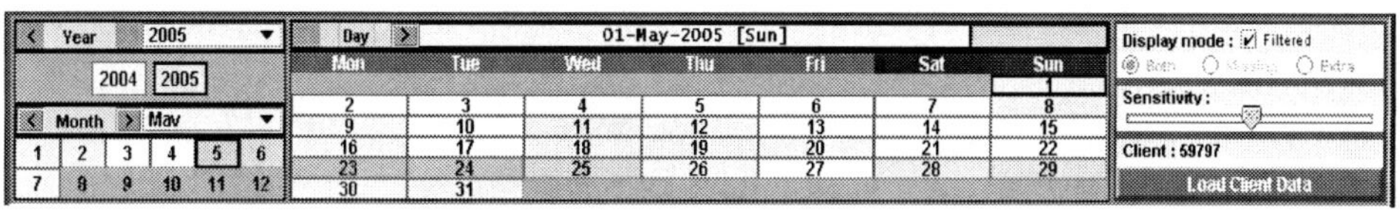

Figure 7: The Calendar View

4.2. B. The Analyses Reporting Views

A number of views provide specific information regarding the well-being status questions discussed earlier. The first daily activity plot displays sensor data and inferred activities of the client on the currently selected day. This is composed of the control panel on the left side and a 24-hour colored plot of data on the right, as shown in Figure 8 (Note that the original view is color intensive). The plot contains three groups of information from the pre-processed sensor data, which are fully listed for selection in the control panel:

1. Activity group - The first group, forming the majority of the view, lists all the individual sensors, for example, front door open/close, bed occupied, kitchen PIR, etc. This first group also contains the 'activity' level (constructed as the

aggregate of all PIR sensor firings in 5 minute periods) and 'silence' (long periods where no data was observed).

2. Location group - The second group lists all the individual PIR sensors. This data is condensed onto one timeline with colored stripes representing the rooms where and when motions were detected.
3. Abstract group - The third group contains the abstracted activities such as ASLEEP, OUT, INACTIVE, VISITOR, and BATH. The VISITOR activity differs from the others in that its color is displayed brighter (toward yellow) as the confidence for a visitor being present increases. The confidence level is a result of applying fuzzy reasoning as described in detail in Section III. In addition to ASLEEP, there are also the minor activities of DRIFTING, WAKING, and STIRRING events that indicate the periods before, after and disturbances during the sleep periods respectively. These and all other activities are inferred by analyzing the data from the relevant sensor activity group.

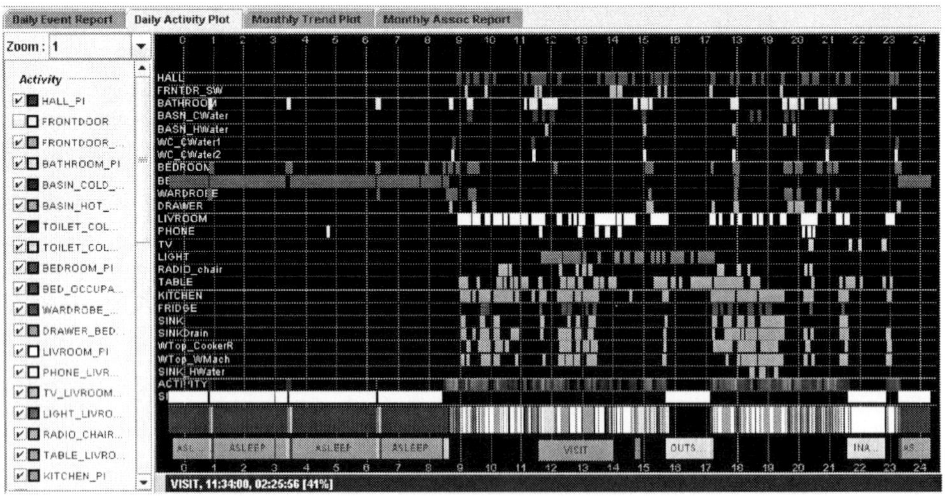

Figure 8: Daily Activity View

Other important views are used to display changes of the well-being related values such as sleeping, eating, going out, and having visitors. Original values, their moving average, plus changes in trend can all be shown. To make the system user-friendly, analyses are chosen from a list of questions relating to well-being and derived from the well-being model of the Domain Specific Modeling project within the centre.

5. Conclusions

The aim of this telecare project is to deliver a solution whereby a care-giver can constantly observe the behavior of a person remotely, changing the provision of assistance to a more efficient and less intrusive on-demand service. Intelligent data analysis is used to monitor the long-term well-being of vulnerable persons living at home, with primarily trend analysis, pattern discovery, and association analysis applied to capture comprehensive information about a person's daily activities. However, in order to provide activity specific reports to the care professional, the large amount of data collected by the sensors installed in the home of the client must be pre-processed and converted into abstract activity information (i.e. sleeping, social interaction, eating, ...etc).

There are a number of factors that can cause uncertainty and ambiguity in the process of obtaining the abstract activity information. First of all, the sensors were designed to be completely non-intrusive which excludes the use of any form of tagging for personal identification. This means that there is a degree of ambiguity in terms of the identity of the person performing an activity, and in terms of the number of people in the home at any one period of time. The second issue is related to the need to restrict the number of sensors used in any one home to a reasonable limit otherwise the cost would be prohibitive. As a result of these factors, it was decided to use fuzzy logic techniques in pre-processing the data and in obtaining the abstract activities.

The analysis of well-being is very challenging, as normal patterns of behavior are difficult to obtain. In addition, what is considered to be normal for one person can be abnormal for another. Moreover, people have a tendency to change the way they do things without necessarily being affected by deterioration in their physical or mental abilities. Therefore interactive and adaptive algorithms are necessary to handle such analysis with the particularities of each individual in mind. Learning algorithms are being introduced to the system in order to handle these issues.

References

[1] R.G. Curry, M. Tinoco, and D. Wardle, "Telecare; Using Information & Communication Technology to Support Independent Living by Older disabled and vulnerable people", Report on behalf of the Department of Health UK, [Online]. Available: http://www.icesdoh.org.uk/downloads/ICT-Older-People-July-2003.pdf.

[2] The Care in the Community Centre Website, www.dticareinthecommunity.com

[3] World Health Organisation, "Active Aging: A Policy Framework", [Online], 2002. http://www.who.int/hpr/ageing/ActiveAgeingPolicyFrame.pdf

[4] B. Majeed, D. Nauck, B. Azvine, and B.-S. Lee, "Intelligent condition monitoring for tele-care systems," The 33rd International Conference on Computers and Industrial Engineering, CD ROM proceeding, Jeju, Korea, Mar. 2004.

[5] R. Kruse, J. Gebhardt, and F. Klawonn, Foundations of Fuzzy Systems. Wiley, Chichester ,1994.

[6] L. Zadeh, , "Soft computing and fuzzy logic", IEEE Software, vol. 11, pp 48—56, 1994.

Promoting Independence for Older Persons with Disabilities
W.C. Mann and A. Helal (Eds.)
IOS Press, 2006

A Community Based Integrated Service Model to Support Adults with Physical Disability Living in the United Kingdom

Suzanne MARTIN[a,1], Christopher NUGENT[b], Jonathan WALLACE[b], Maurice MULVENNA[b], Eileen THOMSON [C], Stephen MATHEWS[C]
[a]*Faculty of Life and Health Sciences, University of Ulster at Jordanstown, UK.*
[b]*Faculty of Engineering, University of Ulster at Jordanstown, UK,* [c] *The Cedar Foundation, 31 Ulsterville Avenue Belfast.*

Abstract. This work describes a 'Smart Home' Service model within the United Kingdom. The community based supported housing scheme accommodates adults with physical disability within their own apartments. These tenants, who had previously lived in a residential facility, are now empowered within the Social Model of Disability to live as autonomously as feasible. User perspectives of autonomous living are reported, enabled by a combination of care packages, environmental design and information and communication technology. A service provider perspective is presented, underpinned by the exploitation of resources (financial or otherwise) from statutory and non-statutory multi-agency involvement. This work reports on an evaluation of the scheme. The strategic context and operational policies at organization level are described as well as service provider and service user perspectives. The applicability of 'Complexity Theory' is considered as a conceptual framework for considering this service model. Complexity Theory facilitates acknowledgment of the inherent dynamics of the system. The dependency on numerous organizations, the connectivity of people and the context of the service are all recognized. This understanding is relevant as service providers move to sustain mainstream Smart Home provision, managing the unpredictability, moving beyond pilot studies.

Keywords. Physical disability, information and communication technology, smart home

Introduction

Social care service providers have historically exploited Information and Communication Technologies (ICT) to support disabled and elderly people at home. Currently a proliferation in the range of technologies and applications is emerging in both literature and mainstream services [2]. In Europe, three key issues have together stimulated the emergence of innovative and dynamic service models that utilize ICT to support the independence and autonomy of disabled people in community settings. These are the expanding role of community care services, the evolution of the social models of disability and a growing recognition of user empowerment [3].

The pace of change is gaining momentum and services traditionally provided within the acute and tertiary sectors are now feasible in the community. In parallel, non-traditional organizational partnerships are emerging which facilitate community service provision in a format which challenges previously established norms. Often a mixed economy of service input is utilized to support disabled and elderly people at home, for example ICT, care packages and environmental adaptation. Service providers and service users are interested in understanding how ICT integrated into Social Care can move towards sustainable mainstreamed services beyond pilot projects.

This work focuses on one such scheme based in Belfast, Northern Ireland. Hillmount Close (Belfast, U.K) is a new, purpose built, supported living, housing scheme for people with complex physical disabilities. Developed in partnership by Cedar Foundation (www.cedar-foundation.org) and Habinteg Housing Association (www.habinteg-ulster.co.uk), the design incorporates 'best practice' in applying housing standards for disabled people, integrating ICT in the form of networked interactive environmental control systems.

The accommodation consists of two apartment blocks, two stories high on a single site. Each block contains two ground floor apartments for wheelchair users and two on the 1st floor for ambulant disabled people. Each apartment is fully networked with the European Installation Bus (EIB). Into this peripherals are connected which can be operated via infra-red signal. These peripherals when activated carry out functional tasks for the tenants that they are not physically able to perform. These include automatic door access, window and blind control, heating controls, lighting control and devices to access entertainment i.e. radio and TV. Tenant's end user device specification for activation of peripherals varies according to ability.

The integrated system enables combination scenario's to be utilized by the individual. As an example on leaving the apartment the system will check that all windows and doors are closed, and relevant electrical items turned off. Personal care and support is commissioned on an individual tenant basis via Government funding i.e. Health and Personal Social Services and delivered by Cedar Foundation care staff. A variety of funding agencies are exploited to financially facilitate the tenure with the Housing association. This scheme became fully operational during July 2003 when the first tenants moved in. Hillmount Close offers a viable alternative to institutional care and potentially a transitional living option for tenants.

Detailed results of Living and working at Hillmount Close have been reported at ICOST 2005 [4]. This work reports on a much higher level of abstraction, considering the wider evaluation exploring the totality of the service model required to sustain tenants at Hillmount Close.

1. Methodology

This work was undertaken in two separate components by two different investigators, who collaborated on the overall approach to data gathering, and the final document synthesis for the funder. A combined methodology of qualitative and quantitative components was deployed. One investigator gathered data using focus groups for tenants and individual interviews with staff members. External consultations were also held with relevant key stakeholder i.e. South and East Belfast Health and Personal Social Services Trust, Northern Ireland Housing Executive and the Centre for Independent Living. The second investigator, met individually with tenants, in their apartments and staff members in their offices.

1.1. Study aim

The overall aim of the study was to evaluate the project as a model of practice for providing sensitively adapted accommodation and as a dynamic care support package which recognizes the individual lifestyle of each service user.

1.2. Study Objectives

- To explore the role of organizational partnership's during Scheme development.
- To investigate the processes of tenant assessment and selection.
- To reflect on the identification and delivery of training to prepare the tenants for independent living.
- To reflect on the identification and provision of training to staff to facilitate independent living.
- To investigate the SMART Home technology and the interactive environmental control systems in facilitating independent living of people with complex disabilities.
- In terms of the commissioning phase, to establish the effectiveness of the Housing Scheme against the core values of Cedar Foundation.
- To investigate the internal and external systems for quality assuring the effectiveness and efficiency of the project.

2. Key Findings

The development at Hillmount Close has been achieved through a well planned and structured operational direction, which evolved from the Cedar Foundation's Strategic Review of Accommodation Services, in May 2000. As a model of practice, Hillmount Close, embodies the three core principles that underpin the provision of accommodation services as identified in the Cedar Foundation's Strategic Review. These are independent living, equal opportunities and user involvement.

This is evidenced by the testimony of the tenants, operational policies and activities like the tenants user forum. Promoting effective user involvement is one of the key themes of the Cedar Foundation's 3-year Strategic Plan 2005 – 2008. Partnership working with service users is central to the organization's culture and business processes. The Cedar Foundation User Forum plays a key role in informing and influencing service development at both a strategic and operational level.

A multi-agency approach was essential to bring the idea of supported housing from vision to reality. Statutory and non-statutory providers were essential contributors to drive forward the development and establish a solid base of good practice that is in keeping with current strategic policy and legislation. Agencies included Healthcare Providers, Housing Associations, Supporting People Funding. A new relationship was established as the disabled adults acquired tenure of apartments rather than passive recipients of accommodation.

The provision of Electronic Assistive Technology within Hillmount Close supports a unique opportunity of community living for people who had previously been within residential or hospital care. The technology is integrated into the physical environment and merges seamlessly into the functional activity of individual tenants.

In general there is a high level of satisfaction among tenants with the built environment, which has been developed to offer a high quality living experience tenants although there were some unanticipated limitations arising from the inheritance of the existing site and footprint of the building. Facilities are not shared, so tenants enjoy high levels of privacy and autonomy. An important feature of the Hillmount Close development is that the apartments are of sufficient size to allow tenants to socialize and meet in each others apartments when they wish to do so.

The process of assessment and selection of tenants can be judged as having been successful for two main reasons. First, all those who were selected as tenants at the outset have remained in the project with the exception of one tenant who has now moved on to a more independent living situation.

Tenants report feeling a high level of independence and autonomy in their everyday lives. They perceive themselves to have control over everyday lifestyle decisions. Tenants' control over their individual environments is maximized through the use of the electronic assistive technology for those who require it. Care and support is provided in a highly individual manner through individual person centered planning based on individual need and not on a group basis. The relationship of tenants with health and social care providers is changing to that of commissioner of care services within their own home.

Successful implementation of the Hillmount Close Scheme has required a very broad base of expertise from individuals within a range of organizations for example, community care provision, provision of supported living funds, rehabilitation, integrated housing development, housing management and the design and development of electronic assistive technology.

The initial eighteen months of operation at Hillmount Close have been a period of transition and change for both staff and tenants. The move to working and living in a scheme that is operating a new model of practice involves participating in a highly dynamic environment where experiential learning and reflection is as important as formal training. Diversity and flexibility of care staff skills are required to move responsively from one task to another and from one tenant to another. Staff acknowledged both the stresses and satisfaction involved in supporting the independent living of adults with complex needs, recognizing both the benefits for tenants and for ongoing professional development to be gained from working within this dynamic innovative model of care.

The transition to this model of practice essentially involved a cultural change, requiring a broad approach that included changes at all levels in the organization from high level statements of values and principles and changes in professional language and terminology through to changes in virtually every aspect of day-to-day practice to reflect the new model of delivery. The location of staff and managers on the Hillmount Close site has been fortuitous in this regard as the close working proximity has been a useful means to ensure the maximum opportunity for infusion of experiential learning.

Quality is assured by robust operational systems within the Cedar Foundation that are constantly kept up-to-date through ongoing review and formal accreditation, which is further reinforced by the involvement of managers in practice development within the sector. The Foundation is committed to continuous improvement as evidenced by the entire organization achieving ISO 90012000 registration in 2005 as well as holding a wide range of quality awards. These include the Mark of Excellence, the European Quality in Rehabilitation Mark, Charter Mark and 6 prestigious National Training Awards. The Foundation has also been an Investor in People since 1997.

3. Conclusion

The Cedar Foundation, established in 1941, is a voluntary organization whose mission is to deliver a range of services which empower and support adults, children and young people with physical disabilities and acquired brain injury to be fully included in their communities.

Within this portfolio Hillmount Close is a unique facility which has integrated ICT, environmental design and care provision developing a holistic, tenant driven service model. This model is multi-agency requiring strategic partnerships across a range of statutory and non-statutory organizations. This approach has been successful in providing a mainstream service, beyond pilot project.

Hillmount Close is sustainable and supporting adults with disabilities, previously in residential care, to live autonomously in the community. The research demonstrated that the Cedar Foundation have successfully developed a model of practice, which integrates environmental design and care provision in a dynamic way to support the individual lifestyle of tenants.

During this research an appreciation of the complexity inherent within such provision became apparent. Cross organizational collaboration was essential, working with multiple systems, dealing with emergent properties of the new service and both intended and unintended consequences. Connectivity was essential between the tenants and a range of staff from a variety of places, all within the new context of Hillmount Close.

For this reason 'Complexity Theory' and systems thinking in general may be a reasonable framework within which to address future similar Smart Home developments [5].

Acknowledgments

Appreciation is extended to the Cedar Foundation for funding this work. The contribution of Evelyn Gilliland is also acknowledged and greatly appreciated.

References

[1] Cedar Foundation, 2005. *Evaluation of Hillmount Close Supported Living Scheme.* Belfast: Cedar Foundation.

[2] Curry, R.G., Tincon, MT., Wardle, R., *Department of Health July 2003,* Telecare:Using Information and Communication Technology to Support Independent Living by Older, Disabled and Vulnerable people.

[3] Hudson, B., 1999. *The Changing Role of Social Care.* Great Britain: Athenaeum Press, Gateshead, Tyne and Wear.

[4] Martin, S., Nugent, C., Porter-Armstrong, A., 2005.User Perspectives: Living and Working within a Smart Home Environment. *In:* S, Giroux,. H, Pigot,ed. *ICOST2005 From Smart Homes to Smart Care,* 3rd *International Conference on Smart Homes and Health Telematics* Sherbrooke Canada, July 2005. Amsterdam: IOS Press, pp33-41.

[5] Whiteford, G., Klomp, N., Wright-St. Clair, V., 2005. Complexity Theory: Understanding Occupation, Practice and Context. *In:* Whiteford, G., Wright-St.Clair, V., eds. *Occupation and Practice in Context.* Australia: Eslevier, pp 3-15.

Promoting Independence for Older Persons with Disabilities
W.C. Mann and A. Helal (Eds.)
IOS Press, 2006

Ageing People in Ireland: A Survey Perspective on Technology in the Home

Sinéad MCEVOY[a,1], Maurice MULVENNA[c], Rodd BOND[b], Chris NUGENT[c], Mary SHAPCOTT[c]
[a]*Health Services Executive-North East Area, Co. Louth, Ireland*
[b]*Dundalk Institute of Technology, Co. Louth, Ireland*
[c]*School of Computing and Mathematics, University of Ulster, Northern Ireland*

Abstract: The Irish population aged 65 years and over is increasing and it is predicted that this trend will accelerate over the next 30 years. Projections highlight that those aged 65 and over will number 0.5million by 2011, an increase of 26% representing 14% of the population. In order to anticipate the needs of this increasing segment of our population, a survey of ageing people's needs in Ireland was commissioned. The overall aim of the survey was to determine the needs and requirements of ageing people with respect to assistive technologies in the home. The survey found that a majority of ageing people were willing to embrace the use of technology which would enable them to age in place. However, while acknowledging the benefits of technology and the automation of systems and functions, respondents were concerned that human interaction may be replaced by technical systems over which they would have no control. Furthermore, such technologies must be non-intrusive, failsafe, affordable, easy-to-use and their use must be ethical.

Keywords. Aging, technology, information and communication technology

1. Background

Our global population continues to grow and within this, the percentage of ageing is also increasing. We now face the challenge of healthcare service initiatives driven by the goals of individual autonomy and quality of life. At a European level, during 2002, it was estimated that between 12-17% of the total population was represented by the ageing. These demographical changes will inevitably pose increased problems for social security and healthcare systems.

In Ireland, the population aged 65 years and over is also increasing and it is predicted that this trend will accelerate over the next 30 years. Projections highlight that those aged 65 and over will reach 520,000 by 2011, an increase of 26% and will represent 14% of the total population. Currently the needs of this cohort place a huge financial, medical and social care burden on the relevant agencies that provide services. It is estimated that between the years 2000 and 2050, public health expenditure for acute healthcare will rise from 5.9% to 8.2% of Ireland's Gross Domestic Product (GDP).

We are faced with the challenge to increase the quality of care for increasing numbers of ageing people while reducing healthcare costs. However, healthcare is currently optimised for treating disease and traditionally innovation has been in the area of clinical and pharmaceutical advances. The challenge for providers of healthcare is to devise processes, which optimise wellness incorporating, health promotion, compliance with healthcare intervention and caregiver support. Non-intrusive technologies must become a part of the everyday lives of ageing people empowering them to take greater responsibility for their own health and social well-being. By shifting the balance of healthcare towards individuals in their own environment it may be possible to decrease overall health costs in the long-term. By providing the ageing person with health information, which is timely, accurate and supports self-management, the ageing can expect to live longer and fuller lives. This notion of a personal health system must also reduce the burden of additional workload currently placed on caregivers.

This change in service delivery to accommodate the emerging demographic landscape has large-scale implications for the redevelopment of healthcare infrastructures and their service provision. Inevitably this results in shifting the allocation of resources from tertiary-care institutions towards the preventative management at the primary care level, as well as delivering services to individuals in their own home environment where they are likely to be most cost-effective [8]. Resulting services and infrastructures will primarily focus upon the inclusion of socially disadvantaged people into today's society. This is a complex scenario which can be addressed by the correct balance of the introduction and utilisation of Information and Communication Technologies (ICT) and the services they facilitate, to ensure that all citizens benefit from the information society.

2. Implications of Using ICT

The primary aim of service provision, or any intervention, should be to promote wellness and independence. Advances in medicine and technology have made many fundamental improvements in many areas of healthcare resulting in better management of multiple pathologies and chronic diseases thereby potentially increasing life expectancy. As people grow older, their need for support in the home environment increases. Evolving models of service provision must provide a balance between the technological solutions offered and the needs for support in conjunction with the health needs of people. Efficient systems should consider a person-centred approach as opposed to a service-centred one. The needs of people very often emerge from the difficulties and risks encountered at home in their daily living. Rather than focusing solely on the health concerns of people, we must consider the person as a living human being in a social and geographic environment.

Technology has the potential to change lives, in general for the better and has contributed to fundamental improvements in many areas of our lives including communications, healthcare, transportation and leisure activities. For ageing people to benefit from the advances that technology brings it is essential that systems are designed with their capabilities and limitations in mind, that proper training is provided, and that the needs of the ageing users are considered in the development of future technologies.

New technologies are only as successful as they are easy to use by all members of the user population. Efforts to reach ageing consumers are often hampered by a lack of understanding of the abilities, requirements and preferences of this population. Many computer-based systems have been designed with little regard for the potential ageing adult users [10]. Dewsbury et al. highlight that designing assistive technology solutions for ageing people is fraught with problems due to the number of agencies involved [3]. These problems are compounded by the lack of understanding, which can exist between the diverse ranges of professionals involved in the provision of such services. Despite these challenging factors, Connell and Sanford, state that technological interventions can reduce difficulty in activities of daily living, enhance independence, safety and security for ageing adults and reduce the burden of care for caregivers. In the long run, environmental interventions can be cost effective if they allow elders to remain in their own homes as opposed to relocation to nursing homes [2, 7]. In addition to cost benefits, extending the time for which elders remain in their own homes has the additional benefit of maintaining their perception of independence.

The current and future needs of the ageing population must be researched and examined, the overall aim being to promote collaboration between all agencies ensuring an integrative approach to the delivery of services incorporating health, welfare and social dimensions thereby enhancing the well-being of this population. Design of such services should also take into consideration the elements of integration with existing practice and also the notions of interoperability with other similar models of care.

Smart homes have provided an opportunity to realise this vision where an environment than can promote levels of independence and increase personal autonomy can be established [6]. Developments in the area have been prolific, ensuring an appropriate balance between technological solutions and service delivery provides a positive experience for the person in their own home environment.

3. Smart Homes

A smart home is designed to offer technological support for the person in their home environment to promote levels of independence and increased personal autonomy. The benefits of a smart home may include the following:

- Increased liveability, comfort and peace of mind;
- Lower expenses and maintenance costs;
- Being able to stay in the home longer, amongst a network of family, friends and familiar neighbours;
- Helping the environment.

The smart home environment should be able to adapt according to how the person interacts with the environment either on a real time basis or over a period of time. Smart home technology offers a viable solution to the aforementioned increasing needs of the ageing by facilitating them to remain as independent as possible and to remain in their own homes. Many studies have highlighted that this is a desire of the ageing rather than being admitted to long-term care settings, as is often the case due to the current lack of alternatives [5, 11]. Nevertheless, Barlow and Venables suggest that design and technology innovations must be matched by new care delivery models [1]. Hence we can consider that the successful uptake of Smart homes is a more complex task asides simply introducing technology into the home environment. The developments must be such that they are extensible and interoperable and support not only the persons within their home, but also their support networks [9].

Smart homes that incorporate electronic sensors, video-monitoring, remote health monitoring and equipment such as movement and fall detectors, door monitors, bed alerts, pressure mats and various alarms (smoke, heat, flood, burglar) can improve patients' safety, security and ability to cope at home. Nevertheless, it is important that the use of smart home technology and services is:

- Ethical: the use of smart home technology must take place under strictly controlled ethics;
- Economical: smart home technology must be cost effective for both the user and society;
- Technological: the smart home systems and services must:
  - be designed to suit to the needs and requirements of the individual;
  - be as unobtrusive as possible;
  - ensure the safety and privacy of the individual.
- Psychosocial: smart home technology must be accepted and easily used by participants.

It is interesting to look forward into the technology future for smart homes and note the findings of Dishman et al. in **Table 1** [4]. This is a listing of some key smart home technologies and their usefulness in supporting ageing in place and independent living.

Table 1. Selected Core Technologies and Their Capabilities [4]

Technology	Values to Aging in Place
Wireless broadband	Anywhere in the home, any device connectivity Rich and multiple streams of health information delivery
Biosensors and bodily diagnostics	Real-time, routine chemical analysis Targeted drug delivery and effects analysis
Activity sensors and behavioral diagnostics	Location, object, and person tracking around the home Regular activity and activities of daily living measurement and assessment
Information fusion and inference engines	Personal baselines and alerts to meaningful deviations Reliable data even from temperamental technologies
Personal health informatics	Central repository for personal and professional health information Tools for easy visualization of long-term trends
Ambient displays and actuator networks	Lightweight ways to notice "okayness" of loved ones Smart home controls of all devices and appliances
Agents, assistants, coaches, companions	Reminding and coaching of activities of daily living that are declining Companionship for intellectual stimulus and support
Adaptive, distributed interfaces	Any device interactivity—do not have to use a personal computer to compute Interface experience personalized for familiarity and function
Remote community and collaboration	Multiple modes and media for communicating across distance Ways of representing and feeling "presence" at lonely times

Dishman makes the interesting point that currently many of the devices that facilitate the services in **Table 1** are designed for use by medical professionals. However, as they become cheaper and smaller, they are more available to the rest of us and are being incorporated into simple household devices, while being inter-connected and embedded into household networks.

4. The 2005 Nestling Technology Survey

In order to prepare for the expected impact of increasing care requirements, a study was commissioned in 2005 covering an area in Dundalk, Co Louth, which is situated in the North-East of Ireland. The overall aim of the study was to determine the needs and requirements of ageing people and their circle of carers prior to the commencement of a major smart housing development planned for Barrack Street, Dundalk. This development is planned under the auspices of the 'Nestling Technology' project, a multi-stakeholder project which consults and shares information with all agencies involved ensuring that requirements for independent safe living in the community setting are met.

A random sample of 100 subjects aged sixty-five years or over was selected from lists of people attending active retirement groups, social clubs and day hospitals in the area, people currently receiving services in the community setting, discharges from the acute hospital setting, ageing people residing in both public and private long stay institutions for no longer than twelve months and ageing people on social housing lists. Clients were contacted by phone and invited to participate in the study. Recruitment only took place following a verbal and written explanation to clients and the signing of written informed consent. Face to face interviews were held in clients' own homes or their current place of residence following arrangement by phone. Clients were under no obligation to participate in the study and were free to withdraw at any time.

The scope of the survey itself was intended to be broad. This current paper only describes the early findings relating to use of technology in the home. It is expected that further analyses of the information collected will lead to relevant findings in other specific areas such as potential impact on service delivery, reductions in care givers burdens and presentation and recommendations healthcare care-related needs for adapting environments.

4.1. The Technological Environment

The specific portion of the survey of interest in the current paper dealt with assistive technology (i.e., adaptations to the physical environment and the use of equipment and ICT, sensors and other devices), which would enable people to age in place. Awareness of assistive technology among participants in the population sample was high. However, the assistive technology, which interviewees were more familiar with were those which dealt with adaptations to the physical environment such as grab rails, level showers and wider doorways. Interviewees were less familiar with information and communications technology, the sensor technologies and remote health monitoring technologies.

Eighty-one percent of those interviewed currently used some form of assistive technology in the home environment. All respondents but one (99%) were amenable to using assistive technology in the future and were willing to be trained in the use of the same. It was noteworthy that only 14% had access to home computers and even smaller numbers (6%) had access to the internet.

The use of assistive technology was considered in a number of different areas to include, home access and security, environmental and appliance controls, movement, activity and fall detectors, medicine/medical management, memory aids and social contacts. These are discussed in the following sections.

4.1.1. Home Access and Security

Home access and security were considered. Within this area the majority (76%) preferred to access their home from the front entrance, while (1%) cited preference for back door access and 23% thought it was important to have access from both the front and back. A large majority of respondents (98%) highlighted that access to a garden was an important feature for them.

Security in the home was an extremely important feature for all ageing clients who reported a particular sense of vulnerability to thieves and vandals. The majority of participants indicated their preference for a security alarm, for having lights turn on automatically on their return home and having the facility to view visitors before opening the front door to them. There were also significant but reduced majorities (between 74% and 96%) indicating a preference for automatic illumination on entry to a room and automated opening and closing of curtains at dawn and dusk.

When respondents were asked to consider their preferred method of unlocking their front door, although none had experienced it, iris recognition was the most popular option (69%). 20% opted for standard key, 4% for a number code, 3% for a smart card and 4% for palm recognition.

4.1.2. Environmental and Appliance Controls

All respondents stated that control of their environment from a heating, lighting and ventilation perspective was very important both in terms of reducing financial running costs and being environmentally friendly. Nevertheless, participants expressed the concern that in the environment where things were becoming increasingly automated they would also like to have manual control over these amenities.

With regard to detectors; smoke, flood, fire and burglar systems were considered as very important features in the home for the majority (99%). In addition to this, 99% of respondents felt that sensors in the home to control electrical appliances and different systems such as water were essential for personal safety.

4.1.3. Personal Detectors and Medical Management

All respondents were agreeable to their movements and activities being continuously monitored in the home in the interests of their own safety and welfare. It was explicitly stated by all respondents that this should only take place with their consent when the need arose, otherwise, it would be considered as an invasion of privacy. An external agency (61%) was the preferred choice for the monitoring of these movements, followed by family (36%). The remaining options included friends (1%) and healthcare personnel (2%).

A high proportion (96%) took prescribed medication on a daily basis and stated that where the need arose it would be beneficial for them to have a system in place to ensure they were taking the right medication at the right time. In addition to this those (53%) who had their vital signs (blood pressure, blood gases, oxygen saturation and blood glucose levels) measured on a regular basis favoured a system being in place whereby these signs could be monitored at a remote site with the aim of detecting irregularities at an early stage, obtaining early intervention and preventing acute hospital admission.

4.1.4. Memory Aids

Eight percent of respondents had a diagnosis of Alzheimer's disease and the remaining respondents were very aware of the debilitating effects of dementias and almost all knew of someone who suffered from memory problems. All but one of the participants were in favour of memory aids being installed in the home environment to enable them to remain at home should their memory fail. Participants were asked in what form they would like memory aids/prompts and the overwhelming majority (93%) stated a speaking voice. Results are shown in Table 2.

Table 2. Types of Memory Aids Preferred by Clients

Memory Aid	N (%) (Clients N=100)
Speaking voice	93(93)
Telephone call	2(2)
Light signal	1(1)
Message on television screen	1(1)
Message on computer	2(2)
Not applicable	1(1)
Total	100(100)

4.1.5. Past-times and Social Contacts

Participants were questioned on how they spent their free time. This information is presented in Table 3. A large percentage of the sample watched television and listened to the radio with many finding that this was the only way they had to spend their free time. Although, only a small proportion of respondents had access to a computer (14%) and the internet (6%) they did realise that this would increasingly become the mode of communication in the future.

Table 3. Activities in which interviewees spent their free time

Activity	N (%) (Clients n=100)
Sedentary	65(65)
Active	8(8)
Both	27(27)
Total	100(100)

When asked how they would like to stay in contact with family and friends using technology the majority (92%) stated video-conferencing and the preferred method for interacting with the computer was by voice (60%). Participants stated that enhanced acoustics (65%) and magnified visual displays (30%) were additional features required to make technology user friendly.

5. Summary of Key Findings of Nestling Technology Survey

In summary, 100 people were interviewed and qualitative data was obtained regarding the use of technology. The original sample was varied and consisted of those who were living independently in the community, those who were being cared for by family members in the community and those who were residing in long-term care facilities. It was the expressed wish of the majority (97%) to remain in their own homes even though a high proportion (44%) felt isolated in their own homes. For many there where multiple physical barriers in the home environment associated with baths and showers, the toilet, stairs, access to and from the house, the risk of falls and accidents and difficulty in performing routine daily tasks such as dressing and grooming, hygiene, preparing meals and shopping.

With regard to assistive technology, the majority of the sample was both aware of assistive technology and amenable to using it to enable them to remain in their own homes. All interviewees were familiar with home adaptations to the physical environment; however, they were less familiar with ICT and sensor technologies. Only 14% had access to computers with only 6% of these having access to the Internet. The predominant types of technology currently used were burglar alarms and personal pendant alarms. Despite this, ageing people were willing to embrace new technologies with the potential to promote aging in place.

Ageing people were concerned that in the technological environment where things are becoming increasingly automated, the use of technology could possibly result in a substitute for human interaction. Nevertheless, the use of technology was favoured for increasing security in the home environment and included the following measures:

- Security alarms;
- Automatic turning lights on and off when arrival at home and on entry to a room;
- Automatic opening and closing of curtains at dawn and dusk especially during periods of absence;
- Facility to view visitors at door prior to opening door to them.
-

Control of the environment using technology (heating, lighting, ventilation) was favoured from the point of view of reducing running costs and being environmentally friendly. The use of technology to control the environment would also serve to reduce human labour costs (home support services), as functions would be automated.

The use of fall detectors and movement detectors were accepted as methods of ensuring personal safety; however, it was stipulated that these measures should only be used where the need arises and with the consent of the ageing person and/or their carers.

Ageing people who very often had no close relatives or friends living nearby agreed that an external agency at a remote site should monitor movements whereas others who had family in the vicinity preferred them to monitor their movements.

Remote medical management (telecare) was favoured in that problems would be detected and diagnosed early, intervention commenced and the trauma, often associated with admission to healthcare settings avoided. In addition, this was seen to possibly prevent frustrating visits to doctors' surgeries and out-patient departments where very often physical environmental barriers, lack of suitable public transport and physical frailty make this difficult.

Systems to ensure that the right medication was being taken at the right time were seen to be advantageous as many people suffered multiple pathology and took numerous medications on a daily basis.

Memory aids were also deemed to be of benefit in certain instances with reminders in the form of a speaking voice being favoured.

6. Recommendations & Conclusions from Nestling Technology Survey

Following analysis of the survey it has been possible to present a number of technological recommendations. Technology must be unobtrusive, non-intrusive, failsafe, affordable, easy to use and its use must be ethical. Where there is a possibility of the ageing person's privacy being invaded the consent of the ageing person must be obtained where possible. The use of technology must not replace human interaction. Technology should be used where it:

- Promotes and maintains functional independence of the ageing person, via the automation of functions, for example, turning on/off lights, taps and electrical appliances, opening and closing curtains;
- Promotes cost savings via heating, lighting and ventilation settings in the home;
- Enhances safety in the home environment and the personal safety of the ageing person (burglar alarms, smoke, flood and fire detectors, and facility to view visitors before opening the door to them, fall and movement detectors, and systems to ensure they are taking the right medication at the right time and memory aids where necessary to enhance cognitive ability).
-

A high prevalence of falls was reported among ageing people in the community. Almost half of the ageing people surveyed (47%) possessed personal pendant alarms, however, compliance with the use of these alarms was poor and reasons cited for this were that they were not user friendly, they were not cosmetically pleasing and false alarms were reported to annoy other people.

The challenge for healthcare providers is to introduce appropriate technologies that support people, in this case ageing people. The conclusions from this study indicate that assistive technologies are perceived by ageing people to have the potential to promote ageing in place. Nevertheless, ageing people must be assured that they are in control of the technical environment, not vice versa. These technologies must be unobtrusive, non-intrusive, failsafe, affordable, easy to use and their use must be ethical. Where there is a possibility of the ageing person's privacy being invaded the consent of the ageing person must be obtained. The use of technology must not replace or be seen as a substitute for human interaction.

References

[1] Barlow J and Venables T (2004). Will Technological Innovation Create the True Lifetime Home? Housing Studies. Vol 19, No. 5: 795-810.
[2] Connell BR. and Sanford JA. (1997) Individualising home modifications recommendations to facilitate performance of routine activities. In Lanspery S, and Hyde J Staying put: Adapting the places instead of the People. (pp.113-147) Amityville, NY: Baywood Publishing.
[3] Dewsbury GA. Taylor BJ. And Edge HM. (2002) Designing dependable assistive technology systems for vulnerable people. Health Informatics Journal Vol 8 104-110.
[4] Dishman, E., J.T. Matthews, and J. Dunbar-Jacob, Everyday health: Technology for adaptive aging, in Technology for Adaptive Aging, R. Pew and S. Van Hemel, Editors. 2004. p. 179-204.
[5] Garavan R, Winder R, McGee H. (2001) Health and Social services for Older People (HeSSOP). Consulting older people on health and social services: A survey of use, experiences and needs. National Council on Ageing and Older People.
[6] Helal, S., Winkler, B., Lee, Ch., Kaddourah, Y., Ran, L., Giraldo, C. and Mann, W. (2003): Enabling Location-Aware Pervasive Computing Applications for the Ageing, Proceedings of PerCom 2003 - 1st IEEE Conference on Pervasive Computing, Fort Worth, Texas.
[7] Lanspery S. Callahan JJ. Miller J and Hyde J. (1997) Introduction: Staying put. In Lanspery S, and Hyde J Staying put: Adapting the places instead of the People. (pp.1-22) Amityville, NY: Baywood Publishing.
[8] Nugent, C. and J. Augusto, Management and analysis of time-related data in internet-based healthcare delivery, in Clinical Knowledge Management: Opportunities and Challenges, R. Bali, Editor. 2005. p. 33-51.
[9] Ranganathan A. and Campbell, RH. Supporting tasks in a programmable smart home, Proceedings of ICOST2005, pp. 3-10, 2005.
[10] Rogers WA. Meyer B. Walker N. and Fisk AD. (1998) Functional limitations to daily living tasks in the aged: A focus group analysis. Human Factors. 40, 111-125
[11] Ruddle H, O'Donoghue F, Mulvihill R. (1997) The Years Ahead Report: A Review of The Implementation of its Recommendations. Dublin: National Council on Ageing and Older People

W.C. Mann and A. Helal (Eds.)
IOS Press, 2006

Effects of Currently Available Smart Home Technology on Frail Elders

Vidyalakshmi SUNDAR[a,1], Machiko R. TOMITA[a], Kathleen M. STANTON[a]
[a]*Department of Rehabilitation Science, University at Buffalo, Buffalo, NY*

Abstract. A two-year randomized controlled trial to identify effectiveness of smart homes, using X10 technology was conducted, comparing 34 treatment and 44 control home-based frail elders. Despite decline in health, the treatment group maintained their physical and cognitive functional statuses. The majority of smart home users reported great benefits, and recommended it to others. The application of smart home technology to retrofit existing houses will most likely assist elders to continue living in their own home. Choosing X10 technology, this project intended to assess the benefits of SH function in independent living among home-based frail elderly. For this project, both stand alone devices (for window and door safety tied with motion sensors and chimes, and remote control for TV/VCR, radio, and lighting) and computer controlled devices (for lighting, coffee maker, and medication reminder) were used. The purposes of this two-year SH intervention study were to: 1) test the possibility of application of commercially available X10 technology to make existing houses of frail elderly smart; 2) identify the user's subjective evaluation of SH functions; and 3) assess the effectiveness of the combined computer use and SH functions on participants' functional status and depression.

Keywords. Aging, frail elders, smart home, independent living

Introduction

Among persons aged 65 and over in the US, more than half have at least one disability and a third experience severe disabilities that prevent them from caring for themselves [11]. Elders with disabilities are likely to experience functional limitations, dependence on caregivers, depression, loneliness, and/or low self-esteem, which could lead to institutionalization [1]. National health expenditures will rapidly increase as baby boomers reach retirement age. It is of vital importance to find strategies so that older adults can live in their own home independently as long as they wish. One way to cope with these problems may be to use smart home (SH) technology, which allows timed settings of lights and appliances through a computer, security features, and remote control to ensure that older adults are safe and secure at home. SH technologies could possibly prevent falls and injuries that often lead to subsequent institutionalization. Since a SH can be operated though a computer, users may also benefit from use of the SH computer. Computers with Internet capability have the potential to help frail elders in creating a social network that may improve the quality of their life by providing a new connection to the outside world [10]. To date, SHs have been tested in newly built wired or wireless residential houses and in lab settings with state-of-the-art, comprehensive SH technologies. The majority of older adults, however, tends to live in older homes and are not likely to be able to afford the newest

SH technology. Therefore SH technology is needed to retrofit existing homes. The purpose of this study was to explore the possibility of applying commercially available X10 technology to make 49 existing homes of frail older persons smart and test its effectiveness on functional status in older adults with chronic conditions by conducting a randomized controled trial.

1. Background

1.1. Brief History of SH Technology

It has been a quarter century since the idea of SHs was initiated by homebuilders in the US in the early 1980's. The original concept of a SH was that the dwelling would be wired with a single multi-conductor cable that included electric power wires, communication cables for telephone and video, and other conductors that connect appliances and lamps with electronic devices that control the supply and switching of power [9]. The terms "automated house (AH)," and "wired house" have been used. Early homes used X10 technology which was born in 1975. The name "X10" simply indicates the tenth project by a company in Scotland using existing AC wiring to transmit signals to control lights and appliances. When X10 technology was introduced to the US market three years later, the system consisted of a 16 channel command console, a lamp module, and an appliance module. The wall switch, timer and computer interface were then added on. In the 1980's, X10 became the de facto standard for home automation and was commonly used in the SH business. In 1989, the first low-cost, self-installed, wireless security system was introduced. In the early 1990s, a market analysis predicted two categories of SH consumers: the ultra-high-end with systems of $100,000 and up, and the mass market, with systems less than $35,000 that were predicted to flourish in the market. Despite this optimistic anticipation, moderate acceptance in the high market and virtually no acceptance by the mass market occurred. Until recently X10 was still the sole modular system that can be purchased on a low budget [4].

1.2. SH for Frail Elders

Although SH was not developed to support frail elders, studies have been conducted, at several sites to determine if SH could prevent institutionalization. One of the most comprehensive projects in the world is SmartBo, completed in December 2000 by the Swedish Handicap Institute. The word, "Bo" in Swedish means nest. SmartBo is a two-room, ground-floor apartment in a five-story building where computer technology and electronics were utilized for people with mild to severe disabilities to have control over their home environment and to support independence. Smart Bo uses an intelligent building control system called European Installation Bus that uses sensors in electric switches for lights, on and off controls, infra-red (IR) receivers (from remote control devices), entrance doors, doorbells, telephone signals, motion detectors, kitchen windows, water taps, stoves, and even beds. The system controlled all lighting, most electric power outlets, the motorized lock of the entrance door, and motorized blinds, curtains, and window openers. Although standard and readily available products were used, they had to be controlled by people with various disabilities. Therefore, many additions to computers plus recorded speech recognition were used for presentation of information. The computers were wirelessly networked. Some systems contributed to the safety of older adults. When a person leaves the bed at night, dimmed lamps light the way from bedroom to bathroom. If the person does not return to bed after a pre-set time, the caregivers would then be alerted. Regarding older adults, they concluded that it is economical for the individual and society when elderly people can continue living in a safe way in their own homes instead of moving into institutions [5].

In the US, one of the most comprehensive SH for frail elders is found in the Allegheny Hospital McKeesport Aging Project in Pennsylvania. This project created 14 two-bedroom, 1000 square foot ranch homes for older adults to live in for several months to test ideas and concepts of SH. This project was initiated based on comprehensive studies of in-home safety and health surveys of older adults. For home-safety, the findings indicated that there are needs for fall risk-reduction, bathroom accessibility, and improved fire safety, home security, and outside access. For health, the findings indicated need for depression screening, activities of daily living (ADL) assistance, more social contacts, wills/advance directives, and education for prescribed medications and community programs. To meet these needs, a cluster of Senior Smart Houses was planned with the goal of keeping older adults at home longer, safer, and healthier by controlling, monitoring, and optimizing household appliances and systems [3].

1.3. Purpose of the Study

Newer and comprehensive wireless SH is promising and may reduce health costs and improve quality of life for increasing numbers of older adults and their caregivers. However, the cost associated with its actualization often exceeds what they can afford. Many frail elders are economically disadvantaged, yet they do not want to leave the home they are accustomed to. We converted their houses or apartments, utilizing X-10 products for practical and immediate applications. Since there is no research regarding the effectiveness of SH using current available technology, retrofitting existing homes to this date, we conducted a two-year randomized controlled trial on sustainability of independent living at home among home-based older adults with chronic conditions.

The present study posed six research questions:

1. Would frail elders accept the SH, if it is provided to them?
2. Do older adults using SH maintain physical function better than the control group?
3. Do the users of SH maintain cognitive function better than the control group?
4. Do the users of SH experience less depression than the control group?
5. What are subjective evaluations of SH by frail elders?
6. Is the rate of remaining at home for SH residents higher than the control group?

2. Methodology

2.1. Sampling

The participants in this study were selected from Western New York with a consecutive sampling method. The inclusion criteria were: a minimum of 60 years of age, living alone, having difficulty in ADLs or IADLs due to chronic health conditions without cognitive impairment, and having an interest in using a computer. Based on our previous study, the effect size was determined to be medium (d=.53), requiring approximately 46 participants in each group. However, considering a much higher attrition rate for the control group, we randomly assigned 46 older adults to the treatment group and 67 to the control group. At the two-year intervention, there were 34 participants in the treatment group (26% attrition) and 44 in the control group (34% attrition). Over the period of two years, there were 35 losses. The descriptive statistics for the sample is summarized in Table 1 for the treatment and control groups separately.

Table 1. Demographic Characteristics for Treatment and Control Group (N=78)

	Treatment Frequency (%) (n=33)	Control Frequency (%) (n=43)	Difference
Age	Mean and SD 72.0 (6.0)	Mean and SD 75.6 (3.4)	t= -2.527 p<. 05
Gender			NS
Male	4 (11.8%)	5 (11.4%)	
Female	30 (88.2%)	39 (88.6%)	
Race			NS
Black	10 (29.4%)	8 (18.2%)	
Caucasian	24 (70.6%)	36 (81.8%)	
Housing			NS
Own	19 (55.9%)	24 (54.5%)	
Not Own	15 (44.1%)	20 (45.5%)	
Education			NS
LT High S	2 (5.9%)	7 (15.9%)	
High School	8 (23.5%)	19 (43.2%)	
Some college	7 (20.6%)	10 (22.7%)	
BS/BA +	17 (50.0%)	8 (18.2%)	
Illness			
Arthritis	28 (82.4%)	37 (84.1%)	NS
Hypertension	23 (67.7%)	27 (61.4%)	NS
Cataracts	20 (58.5%)	26 (59.1%)	NS
Cardiovascular disease	14 (41.2%)	20 (45.5%)	NS
Foot problem	10 (29.4%)	6 (13.6%)	NS
Circulation problem	9 (26.5%)	17 (38.6%)	NS
Hearing impairment	9 (26.5%)	9 (20.5%)	NS
Hip/Knee fracture	6 (17.7%)	9 (20.5%)	NS
Depression	5 (14.7%)	6 (13.6%)	NS
Osteoporosis	5 (14.7%)	8 (18.2%)	NS
High cholesterol	5 (14.7%)	5 (11.4%)	NS
Cancer	4 (11.8%)	13 (29.6%)	NS
Effects of stroke	4 (11.8%)	7 (15.9%)	NS
Diabetes	4 (11.8%)	14 (31.8%)	p=.037
Asthma	2 (5.9%)	5 (11.4%)	NS
Urinary tract disease	1 (2.9%)	9 (20/5%)	p=.022

2.2. Instruments

The X10 technology was selected for this project for the following reasons:1) Many homes were estimated to be using the products so if problems occurred, there were already identified solutions, 2) Retrofitting is possible; 3) Installation is rather simple even for persons with little experience in SH; 4) Many compatible products are available and most of other SH products can be used with X-10 products; 5) Control of up to 256 lighting and appliances is possible; and 6) Home networking solutions can be integrated with an IBM or compatible computer that is equipped with Windows, 95, 3.1 or NT, and a CD ROM drive.

We utilized an X-10 ActiveHome kit and other modules. The kit included products that can be used with either a remote control or computer software: a 5-in 1-remote control for lamps and appliances using radio frequency, a plug-in 2-prong lamp module and a 3-prong appliance module, a key chain remote, a two-way transceiver module that receives radio frequency commands from remotes to operate lamps or appliances plugged into it, a computer interface that works with the transceiver module to control the on/off timing of lamps and appliances, and the ActiveHome software for Windows. The computer software was for centralized and automated control of electric devices. In addition, stand alone products were purchased including door and window sensors, a motion sensor, a power flash that is an interface between the security system and an alarm (chime), a wall switch and an emergency response system that can be worn or placed in each room connected to a phone line for automatic dialing to several caregivers. Stand alone products worked independently of the remote control or the computer software. The computer remained on all the time for ActiveHome to operate (currently this requirement no longer exits). The monitor could be turned off. Excluding the computer, the cost for SH system was less than $400.

Computer use monitoring software called Boss Everyware was installed into the participant's computer after obtaining a consent form. The software collects information such as the application file name, active window and duration, and saves them to a dbase III+ log file. It has the ability to filter data and export it to other programs such as Excel and text editors. The key logger was always turned off so it was incapacitated to identify information such as addresses and names on e-mail communications and passwords. Every six months, their log files were copied and transferred to the investigator's computer; some of the data was filtered in dbase and then converted to XLS to sort. Time spent in a particular application category is reported for each participant, including ActiveHome operation, games, e-mail, and Internet use.

To measure functional status, five instruments were used: FIM for ADL [2], OARS' IADL [6], Mobility section of Dysfunction Section of Sickness Impact Profile (SIP) [8], CHART Mobility [12] for handicap measure, and Mini Mental State Exam (MMSE) [7]. Except for SIP, higher scores indicate higher functions. The psychometrics of all instruments above have been established. In addition, health status such as number and type of illnesses, number of medications, and use of health institutions and home treatment as well as aide hours were recorded by a monthly interview. The participants' evaluated their computer use and SH functions at the end of two years.

2.3. Procedure

A computer and/or Internet were provided to participants in the treatment group who did not own them along with computer training. After a 2.5 hour home assessment of the participant by an occupational therapist or a nurse who had been trained for research, a computer engineer visited the house/apartment of participants who were assigned to the treatment group. Steps to create SH are available in smart house at http://www.agingresearch.buffalo.edu.

For a participant with arthritis in the fingers or a problem with fine motor control, a trackball rather than a mouse was provided and for some participants with vision impairment, an enlarged keyboard was provided. The initial installation took three to nine hours depending on the size of the dwelling. No house incurred more than $400 for the X-10 products and other necessary materials. After the initial installation, when participants had a problem regarding X-10 products and the PC, a geriatric nurse, specialized in computer education, consulted with them on the phone first, and if the problem persisted, she visited their home to solve the problem. On average, they visited participants' houses five times in the first year and three times in the second year.

Initially all 39 participants in the treatment group had ActiveHome software on a computer and a remote control. In total, 531 X-10 products were installed for 39 participants' houses. Table 2 summarizes the number of participants who used the products initially and at the end of the study. The outcome measures were collected annually by the interviewers and process measures for healthcare utilization were recorded by e-mail for the treatment group and quarterly phone calls from a nurse for the control group.

Table 2. Number of Participates who had accepted Smart House Systems initially (N=39) and over two years (N=34)

Types of Products and problems	Number of participants who used the products initially (Total initial users, % of 39)	Number of products installed initially	Number of participants who used the products originally, at the end of the study (Total initial users, Users after 2 years, Rate between the two figures)		
Computer	39 (100%)	39	34	34	(100%)
ActiveHome software	39 (100%)	39	34	22	(65%)
Lighting	37 (94.9%)	92	34	21	(62%)
Wall switch	12 (30.8%)	14	12	8	(67%)
Remote control	39 (100%)	39	34	23	(68%)
Chime (for security/ medication)	34 (87.2%)	52	34	23	(68%)
Motion Detector	19 (48.7%)	19	19	10	(53%)
Coffee maker	23 (59.0%)	25	23	12	(52%)
Power flash for window/door security	29 (74.4%)	176	29	18	(62%)

2.4. Analytical Scheme

For research question (RQ) 1, acceptance rates were calculated by the ratio of number of in-use SH functions to the number of the installations. For RQs 2 though 4, to measure physical and cognitive functional changes, one-way ANOVAs with contrast between the 1st and the 3rd measurements were used for the treatment group and control group separately after identifying health status decline due to different types of illnesses. For RQ 5, descriptive statistics were used, and RQ6, subjective evaluation of SH functions and a rate of living status were analyzed using Chi-Square and standard residuals for the cell contribution to the significance.

3. Results

The two groups were initially equivalent for all demographic and health characteristics except for age and types of illnesses. The control group was four years older than the treatment group and the control group had more circulation problems in arms and legs, cancer, diabetes, and urinary tract diseases while the treatment group had more foot problems. However, when levels of severity of illnesses were examined, there were no differences between the two groups. Changes in health and healthcare use over two years are presented in Table 3.

Table 3. Changes in health and Healthcare Use over two years (N=78)

	Initial	**2nd Year**	**3rd Year**	**Difference**
Number of Illness	6.6(3.2)	7.0 (3.4)	7.4 (3.4)	(ANCOVA)
Treatment Control	7.0 (2.9)	7.1 (3.1)	7.5 (3.3)	F=.764 for 3rd year
Number of Medication	5.9 (3.1)	6.2 (3.0)	6.8 (3.1)	(ANCOVA)
Treatment Control	7.6 (4.9)	8.1 (5.3)	8.3 (5.0)	F= .412 for 3rd year
		During the 1st year	**During the 2nd year**	**Both years**
Days in hospital				(Cumulative)
Treatment		.68 days	1.44 days	2.12 (2.31)
Control		2.32 days	1.68 days	4.00 (5.38)
Days in skilled nursing home				(Cumulative)
Treatment		0	0	0
Control		.55 days	0	.55 days
Days they went to rehab facilities				(Cumulative)
Treatment		3.26 days	2.85 days	6.11 (9.77)
Control		1.04 days	1.57 days	2.61 (4.61)
Hours for visiting nurse/year				(Mean of the 2 yrs)
Treatment		.47hours	.96 hours	.71 (2.27)
Control		9.84 hours	6.55 hours	8.17 (32.35)
Hours for home health care aide /wk				(Mean of the 2 yrs)
Treatment		2.71 hours	2.88 hours	2.78 (9.41)
Control		.27 hours	.59 hours	.43 (1.92)
Hours for Personal Care Aide/week				(Mean of the 2 yrs)
Treatment		1.94 hours	1.82 hours	1.88 (5.97)
Control		.25 hours	.75hours	.43 (1.92)
PT home visits/year				(Mean of the 2 yrs)
Treatment		1.09 times	1.09 times	1.09 (4.06)
Control		.27 times	.77 times	.52 (2.11)
OT home visits/year				(Mean of the 2 yrs)
Treatment		.65 times	.15 times	.39 (1.83)
Control		0	.23	.01 (.107)
Hours of social worker visits/year				(Mean of the 2 yrs)
Treatment		.09 hours	.26 hours	.18 hours
Control		1.57 hours	1.98 hours	1.77 hours
Hours of case manager visits				(Mean of the 2 yrs)
Treatment		.74 hours	.62 hours	.68 (2.00)
Control		.18 hours	.02 hour	.10 (.51)

RQ 1 - Would frail elders accept the SH, if it is provided to them? Initially all participants (N=39) accepted SH with various functions. They are presented in the second column of Table 2. At the end of two years, 100% of participants were using a computer, but only 65% were utilizing ActiveHome software to control for SH functions. The remote control and chimes were used by 68% of participants, followed by wall switch (67%), power flash for window/door security and lighting (both 62%). The motion detector was utilized by 53% of participants and the coffee maker, 52% at the end of the study. All of them were using at least one SH function.

RQ 2 - Do older adults using SH maintain physical function better than the control group? Changes in physical functional status were identified using four measures. They are summarized in Table 4. FIM Motor did not show any changes for both groups while two other measures showed a significant decline in only the control group. For SIP Movement, the treatment group started with 104.9 and ended with 118.5 (higher score means more disabled) but the change was not statistically significant. The control group started with a better score of 80.9 and ended up worse (119.4) than the treatment group (F=7.12, p<.001). For IADL total score, the treatment group scored 11.9 initially and stayed the same (11.8) for two years while the control group scored 12.3 initially and dropped to 11.9 which was a significant decline showed a significant difference. The treatment group scored 85.9 for the initial assessment, and scored 84.7 at the end of the study. The control group scored 85.6 initially and 78.7 for the 2nd follow-up (F=6.57, p=.002).

RQ3 - Do the users of SH maintain cognitive function better than the control group? Cognitive function was assumed to be related to computer use. On average, participants used a computer about 18 days per month (or 4.5 days/week), spending 36 hours 43 minutes each month (or 9 hours 10 minutes/week). The applications most used in descending order were: game, Internet, browsing, e-mail, word processing, and manipulation of ActiveHome. The participants spent a mean of 109 minutes per month (or 27 minutes/week) for visiting health sites on the Internet.

Changes in cognitive functional status were identified using MMSE and FIM cognition. Both groups maintained MMSE scores over two years but using FIM Cognition, only the control group showed significant decline from 33.7 to 32.8 (F=8.51, p<.001). The results are shown in Table 4.

Table 4. Changes in functional status over two years (N=78)

	Initial	2nd Year	3rd Year	Difference
FIM Motor				
Treatment	78.21(12.02)	78.32 (13.55)	77.94 (14.55)	F=.020
Control	79.95 (5.03)	80.18 (4.51)	79.86 (4.72)	F=.179
SIP Movement				
Treatment	104.85 (84.87)	113.71 (96.15)	118.50 (95.34)	F=.857
Control	80.89 (84.87)	110.30 (92.26)	119.43 (93.67)	F=7.12 **
IADL total				
Treatment	11.91 (2.60)	12.00 (2.43)	11.79 (2.68)	F=.268
Control	12.25 (1.94)	12.34 (2.12)	11.86 (2.36)	F=3.177*
CHART Mobility				
Treatment	85.9 (18.8)	84.26 (20.75)	84.74 (21.73)	F=.265
Control	85.6 (17.0)	83.62 (19.98)	78.70 (21.77)	F=6.567**
MMSE				
Treatment	29.74 (.75)	29.68 (.77)	29.71(.72)	F=.094
Control	29.43 (.97)	29.57 (.90)	29.34(.15)	F=.692

FIM Cognition				
Treatment	34.03(1.82)	34.03 (1.93)	34.12 (1.81)	F=.275
Control	33.73(1.78)	32.75 (2.35)	32.82 (2.38)	F=8.51***
Depression				
Treatment	10.18 (8.75)	8.59 (9.36)	9.38 (8.74)	F=.694
Control	1.02 (10.82)	9.43 (9.55)	10.52 (11.13)	F=.788

*<.05
**<.01
***<.001

RQ4 - Do the users of SH experience less depression than the control group? Both groups were not depressed using CES-D initially, and over two years they maintained the status quo.

RQ5 - What are subjective evaluations of SH by frail elders? The question of SH evaluation was addressed only for the treatment group. For Importance of the computer, at the end of the 1st year, 26.5% answered "Very important" and 44.1% said "Somewhat important," and at the end of the 2nd year, the answers were shifted toward very positive: 82.4% reported "Very important" and 14.7% said "Somewhat important." Reports of satisfaction with SH were sought at the end of the two years. Among 34 participants, 76.5% reported they benefited from SH "a great deal" and 20.6% said "some," 50% said SH improved their daily life "A great deal," 20% "some," and 30% answered "Not;" 53% reported they gained confidence in dealing with health /physical problems "A great deal," 35% said "Some" and 12% "Not;" when we asked whether SH helped in understanding ADL problems, 44% said "A great deal," 26.5% said "Some" and 23.5% answered "No." Finally, 91% said they would recommend the SH system to others and 6% said "No."

Of the 31 participants who recommended the SH system, 28 people gave specific reasons. The most frequent reason given was "security" by 14 (50%), 8 (28.6%) said "safety," "easy access to lights" by 4 (14.3%), and 2 (7.1%) stated comfort. Among eight participants who did not recommend the SH system, nine reasons were provided. Two people (22.2%) each said "bad experiences," "erratic (TV remote and lighting)," and "the system is not working." One each (11.1%) said "too many problems," "not very reliable'" and "due to hearing problem, security chime is hard to hear." Regarding the impact of computer use including ActiveHome, no one indicated a negative impact. The highest rate was found in knowledge gain (in general) indicated by 33 participants (84.6%). Twenty eight (71.8%) said it affected mental health such as more mental stimulus and less depression, 26 (66.7%) reported increased socialization, 23 (59.0%) said security, 17 (43.6%) each said health and wellness.

RQ6 - Is the rate of remaining at home for SH residents higher than the control group? Using Pearson Chi-Square, the two groups were significantly different (p=.043) in terms of their living status: 80.4% of the treatment group were living at own home at the end of the study period while 65.7% for the control group. For the treatment group, 34 (73.9%) were still in the study, 6 died (13.0%), 1 went to a nursing home (2.2%), 3 quit due to illness (6.5%). For the control group, 44 were in the study (65.7%), 6 (9.0%) died, 3 (4.5%) went to a nursing home, 3 quit due to illness (4.5%) and 10 (14.9%) were not living home for unknown reasons (14.9%).

4. Discussion

This study found that converting an existing home to a smart home using currently available technology was possible for under $400. The level of automation of the home was determined by a participant' desire and the capacity of the house. Once participants learned to use the SH system, they realized the benefits of having it and accepted it. After two years, 52% to 68% of SH functions were in use. The primary reason for nonuse was related to "failure." Participants chose only functions that did not fail and that were most suitable and beneficial for them. Therefore, when we asked the benefit of SH, almost all of them felt it was beneficial. Failure was not necessarily a malfunction of the system but rather the combination of unfriendly features of the X10 and participants' unfamiliarity with the system. For example, when daylight savings time changed the clock on the computer some of the timed lighting features stopped functioning because the clock in the ActiveHome system was no longer synchronized with the computer clock. When the participants were not familiar enough with the settings of the Active Home to make the changes and reset the system, some chose to end the timed lighting and unplug the devices, not knowing that the problem could be easily rectified. Power failures also caused malfunctions with the ActiveHome system, which only required to be reset, but due to unfamiliarity and fear of computer malfunction, they chose to discontinue the device instead. Close to 50% of frail elders chose not to learn how to operate some functions. Among SH features, lighting was the most problematic. Nevertheless, it was one of the most preferred features for safety reasons and the reason for continuity of living at home for some participants. Higher levels of automation may be necessary to make the feature friendlier.

A contrary finding to existing studies is that use of the computer did not make differences in terms of depression. In this study, if participants were diagnosed with depression, they were usually being treated with antidepressants. Also, most of the existing studies that introduced a support system using a computer tested people who were new to the system. In contrast, most participants in the treatment group in this study had been using a computer at least one year. The longer they used the computer; the importance they place on the computer becomes stronger because computer use becomes a part of life.

Another clear study finding is that SH/computer users maintained physical and cognitive functions over two years in contrast to a significant decline among nonusers. Although increased comorbidity usually translates to declines in motor function, for the treatment group, SH systems could have prevented falls and injuries and allowed more independent daily activities. It is difficult to measure what was prevented by use of SH. Falls can occur more frequently among more active older adults than sedentary older adults. A question is whether we can attribute these findings to the effectiveness of SH. Since this study used a randomized controlled design, the findings tend to be supported affirmatively. However, different types of illnesses will develop differently over two years. The illnesses in the control group participants may have affected their functional status more. Age would also be a factor in greater decline, as the control group participants were, on average, four years older than the intervention group. To clarify the effectiveness of SH, therefore, use of homogeneous participants such as those having similar illnesses and age is recommended for future research.

Finally, significantly more SH users continued living in their own homes than nonusers (80% vs. 66%). SH may have prevented an injury and promoted an active life style. Psychologically, feeling secure also may have encouraged frail elders to continue living at home. Creating a SH needs skill, and living in a SH requires patience in learning how to operate SH technologies. Nevertheless, we conclude that retrofitting an older home with smart home technology can be an effective coping strategy for remaining in one's own home, with quality of life for older adults with chronic conditions.

References

[1] Butler, R. N., Lewis, M. I., & Sunderland, T. (1998). Aging and mental health :Positive psychosocial and biomedical approaches (5th ed.). Boston, MA: Allyn & Bacon.

[2] Center for Functional Assessment Research. (1990). Guide for the use of the uniform data set for medical rehabilitation (Version 3.1). Buffalo, NY: CFAR: University at Buffalo.

[3] Computer Science and Robotics, Carnegie Mellon University. (2003). Blueroof Technologies: The development of a non-profit organization devoted to extending elderly independent living. Retrieved June 20, 2004, from http://www-2.cs.cmu.edu/~nursebot/web/course-spring03/BlueroofPresentation.ppt

[4] Driscall, Jr. E. (2004). The History of X10. Retrieved April 11, 2004, from http://home.planet.nl/~lhendrix/X10_hisory.htm.

[5] Elger, G. (2001). SmartBo - A smart houses for people with disabilities. Retrieved May 20, 2004, from http://www.deafblindinternaitoanl.org/review/samrbtbo.htm

[6] Fillenbaum, G. (1988). Multidimensional functional assessment of older adults: The Duke older Americans resources and services procedures. Hillsdale, NJ: Lawrence Erlbaum Associates.

[7] Folstein, M., Folstein, S., & McHugh, P. (1988). Mini-mental state: A practical method for grading the cognitive state of patients for the clinician. Journal of Psychiatric Research, 12, 189-198.

[8] Gilson, B. et al. (1975). Sickness impact profile: Development of an outcome measure of health care. American Journal of Public Health, 65, 1304-1325.

[9] Gross, M. D. (1998). Smart house and home automation technologies. In W. van Vliet (Ed.), Encyclopedia of Housing. Retrieved June 16, 2004, from http://depts.washington.edu/dmachine

[10] Nahm, E. S. (2003). A model of computer-mediated social support among older adults. Dissertation Abstracts International, 64, 1181.

[11] McNell, J. M. (1997). Disabilities affect one-fourth of all Americans: Proportion could increase in coming decades. Census Brief. Retrieved April 22, 2004, from http://landview.census.gov/prod/3/97pubs/cenbr975.pdf

[12] Wolinsky, F. D., Callahan, C. M., Fitzgerald, J. F., & Johnson, R. J. (1993). Changes in functional status and the risks of subsequent nursing home placement and death. Journal of Gerontology, 48(3), S94-101.

Promoting Independence for Older Persons with Disabilities
W.C. Mann and A. Helal (Eds.)
IOS Press, 2006

Privacy Management in Smart Homes: Design and Analysis

Ryan BABBITT [a,1], Johnny WONG[1], Simanta MITRA[1], Carl CHANG[1],
[1]*Department of Computer Science, Iowa State University, Ames, IA*

Abstract. This work addresses the issue of designing for privacy in smart homes. We identify several principles to guide privacy management in smart homes, propose and analyze several general privacy management techniques, and evaluate existing privacy management efforts in ubiquitous computing. We conclude by explaining how existing work is not contextually expressive enough to give inhabitants the level of control they should have over their personal information. The contributions of this work are threefold: an increased understanding of the notions of privacy and designing for privacy within smart homes and the proposal of new solutions to handling privacy related issues within smart homes, and the facilitation of the acceptance of smart home technology into mainstream society.

Keywords. Smart homes, privacy, ubiquitous computing

Introduction

Smart homes aim to provide a living environment that enhances the quality of life of its inhabitants by providing such services as health and safety monitoring, audio, visual, or tactile reminders, and assistance with various physical and mental tasks. Actions that once needed the (costly) expertise of the doctor or the assistance of a worker at the local senior care center now have the possibility of being done in the comfort of home, allowing those advanced in years or those with special needs to empower themselves to live more independent and fulfilling lives as long as possible.

Though such technologies open the doorway to wonderful possibilities for computer-enriched assisted living, they also present ample opportunity for severe privacy violations as the smart home system actively monitors, stores, uses, and releases to outside parties data of a potentially intimate nature about its inhabitants. Information that falls into the wrong hands or is misused can easily be used to embarrass, deface, or coerce inhabitants. It is therefore critical that privacy management be included in early stages of smart home development because, without a satisfactory privacy management scheme, users will feel discomfort and distrust of their homes, resulting in an overall deterioration of the empowering advantages that computer-aided homes.

The remainder of the paper is organized as follows: section 2 provides a background of smart homes, section 3 provides a privacy analysis of smart homes that culminates in the several privacy design principles, section 4 discusses ways to achieve these principles, section 5 discusses related work, and section 6 concludes the paper and identifies our future efforts.

1. Background in Smart Homes

As mentioned in the introduction, smart homes seek to automate living environments by incorporating different types of sensing devices, acting devices, and controlling devices into some sort of software architecture. This is done to provide inhabitants with such services as task assistance, memory amplification, status monitoring, and emergency notifications. As this technology evolves, new devices and services become available and old ones are replaced, producing a very dynamic and heterogeneous environment.

To manage this complexity, researchers have proposed various system architectures, which can be classified into three types of frameworks: agent-based frameworks, context-based frameworks, and infrastructure-based frameworks. Agent-based frameworks [9] use software agents and artificial intelligence to provide services to inhabitants, context-based frameworks [21] focus on the gathering and interpretation of contextual information from the environment, and infrastructure-based frameworks [16, 4] emphasize the interoperability and networking of devices and services. These approaches are not solutions to the whole but rather complimentary techniques that when combined can strengthen each other.

They all, however, share a similar flaw in their designs. Namely, they neglect inhabitants' privacy concerns, which is completely unsatisfactory. Smart homes are constructed to collect, analyze, and distribute data of an inherently personal and private nature. This fact undeniably requires smart homes to employ an effective and usable privacy management system. If end users do not trust their smart homes or are not comfortable with the services provided therein, then they will, as a result, participate less in smart home technology or completely reject the assistive benefits it provides.

2. Privacy Analysis of Smart Homes

The last several years have seen a flourish of research in privacy related issues in ubiquitous computing. Before delving into the most recent work, we want to introduce some general privacy principles and discuss their application to smart homes.

Privacy has been broadly stated in colloquial terms as "the right to be left alone" or "the right to select what personal information about me is known to what people", several legal efforts in the late 20th century further defined these concepts of information privacy resulting in what is known as *Fair Information Practices* [1, 2, 8, 14]. The main concepts of these principles are summarized below.

- **Openness and Transparency** - Individuals should know about the existence and content of all records that contain information about them.
- **Individual Participation** - Individuals should have access to those records and have the ability to correct that information if it is wrong.
- **Explicit Consent** - Individuals should unambiguously and purposefully agree to the collection of their data.

- **Collection Limitation** – More data should not be collected than is needed by the current task.
- **Data Quality** - Data should only be collected with a specific purpose in mind and be kept accurate.
- **Use Limitation** - Data should be used only for the purpose for which it was collected by appropriately authorized individuals.
- **Reasonable Security** - The security of data should be proportional to its sensitivity, i.e. more personal data should be kept more secure.
- **Accountability** - Collectors/users of data should be held responsible for their collection and use of data according to the above principles.

Several conclusions can be inferred from these principles and applied to smart homes. First, smart home devices and services should always be known to inhabitants, and they should always be aware of the capabilities of their homes. Second, these devices and services should be explicitly defined in such a way that their purpose(s) and method(s) of data usage, how long the data is needed, the security of the data storage, and any conditions under which the service releases the data are made known. Third, information requests from external entities such as third party systems or guests should also contain this information. Fourth, data owners need be able to specify limitations on the collection and use of their personal data, and either the user or the system on behalf of the user must explicitly consent to every information request for personal data. These requests are granted if and only if the user's policy and service definition do not conflict. These principles do *not*, however, require that data owners make their privacy preferences available to requesting entities or that requesting entities should even have access to the data owner's policies. In fact, an individual's privacy policies should be treated the same way as other personal data because they are inherently private information as well.

Langheinrich [21] further analyzed these principles in with respect to ubiquitous computing concepts and modified them slightly, adding two principles:

- **Anonymity and Pseudonymity** - A data owner's identifying information or actions should not be traced back to the individual or any trusted entity acting on behalf of the individual. That is, services should have fair amount of uncertainty about whom they are serving.
- **Proximity and Locality** - Data owners should only be contacted by services that are immediately pertinent to them to minimize the intrusion caused by notifications and requests. This can be done using any type of spatial, temporal, or other user-defined heuristic.

From the smart home perspective, anonymity and pseudonymity means that entities should not have access to data that is theirs, unless that access is explicitly granted to them by the data's owner. This includes preferences and profile information as well as personal data. However, we also note that much of the functionality of a smart home is based on the identity or profile of its inhabitants and maintaining that anonymity may degrade that inhabitant's quality of service and possibly the quality of service of others in the home as well.

The principle of proximity and locality can be applied to smart homes by limiting the intrusion upon the lives of inhabitants. To avoid burdening the occupants with service announcements or consent requests, the smart home should have a mechanism to allow an occupant to specify the conditions under which he/she is explicitly contacted. The remainder of the time the system should automatically evaluate data requests on behalf of the user, and only alert the user if a problem is detected.

Another insightful analysis by Beckwith [6] adds another facet of privacy called information sensitivity. This concept implies that the very nature of data itself influences its privacy level. That is, more personal data is inherently more private than less personal data. This stands to reason but begs the question: what exactly makes data personal? Ideas proposed by Blaine et al. [7] uphold that aside from the data's nature, its precision, accuracy, and freshness also affect its privacy. That is, the more specific the data gets, the closer the data is to the actual quantity measured, and how recent the data is will all affect its privacy-level. Thus, when users define their privacy policies, they should be able to include these three notions in their preferences.

Another aspect of privacy that we have not yet mentioned is that privacy is a dynamic notion; it is inherently subjective and varies across individuals and time. This means that different occupants will have different privacy needs in different situations. Consider the following scenario. Two individuals named Alice and Bob are taking medicine for a degenerative memory disease. Alice on one hand has come to terms with this fact and is not bothered if anyone knows this, or how they use this information. However, Bob is not as comfortable as Alice and wishes that only family members know this about him and that the data is otherwise used only for the medical purpose of his treatment. But what if Bob joins a support group that then boosts his confidence to Alice's level and changes his view of his situation? His privacy requirements will then change as well. Thus, occupants need to be able to define their *own* privacy preferences and be able to freely *change* them at any point in time. This means the system also needs a mechanism to support changes in a user's privacy policy.

Until now we have only observed that an individual's privacy requirements *can* change but have not discussed *what* makes them change, i.e. what states, conditions, events, or situations cause an individual to view his/her private information differently. This notion of situation-based preferences is called context and is defined more formally in software systems as "the circumstances or situations in which a computing task takes place" [23]. Let us illustrate this concept with another brief example. Consider another individual named Carol, and suppose that under normal circumstances she does not want anyone to have access to her location information. However, Carol also wants her family and doctor to be able to find her quickly in the event of an emergency, which will require the use of location information. She treats the same data differently in different contexts. Thus, any privacy management system must also include contextual information in its policy specifications. We further investigate what comprises smart home context in section 4.2 and now offer a summary of our privacy analysis and present several design goals for smart home privacy management.

- **Total Control** - Because privacy is subjective, users know their privacy needs best and should be given the opportunity to fully specify the management of their data in all situations. Users also need to be able to change their preferences.
- **Equal Opportunity** - Different users should be given equal expressive ability and equal chance to manage their own data. Giving some inhabitants more expressive (and thus more effective) privacy policies than others will allow

some inhabitants better control over their data, which inherently unfair to some inhabitants and something that should be avoided.

- **Context Inclusion** - Because privacy is so situational, providing total control of personal information to an inhabitant requires that the context surrounding the data request should be somehow contained in an inhabitant's privacy policy.
- **Non Intrusion** - This principle means that users should be notified of services or data requests only when necessary and that the system should minimize the work for inhabitants during policy creations and validations.

3. Towards Privacy Management Goals

Having identified our main privacy management goals, we now propose and discuss possible approaches to meet these goals.

3.1. On Realizing Total Control and Equal Opportunity

To empower an inhabitant to achieve total control over personal information, we look for all the opportunities in the system during which a user has the ability to exert some restriction on his/her data. Generally speaking, any piece of data has three such opportunities. They are

- Data Collection
- Data Storage
- Data Access

3.1.1. Data Collection Policies

Users can be empowered during data collection by allowing them to decide what types of personal data are collected under what circumstances. This means that users control whether or not data is available to the smart home, which will most likely be done by controlling when information gathering services are operating. This applies to services that read data directly from sensors as well as services that generate information by aggregating lower level data sources. Ultimately, the idea behind data collection policies is that if the inhabitant does not feel comfortable with the data existing, it should not be in the system.

The obvious major drawback of this approach is that the quality of the service provided by a smart home depends heavily on the data contained in it. So a service needing data that is not available may not operate as well or may possibly even fail. This behavior may then propagate through the system as other services that depended on the first service fail. This problem will be made worse if data dependencies in a system are not known because failures will seem to randomly cascade through the system. However, we can counteract this by requiring services to formally specify their definitions, especially their data dependencies, and using some sort of monitoring mechanism to detect and correct service failures.

3.1.2. Data Storage Policies

Users can be empowered by data storage policies by determining how long personal information is stored in the system as well as deciding the accuracy and precision at which it is stored. One possible implementation of a data storage policy might allow data to exist only as long as the requesting service needs it. However, this would require any application that needs time intervals of data to continuously request for and store the current data in order to have access to it later. This would not be efficient in systems that have many profile-based services.

Another, possible data storage policy would be to collect and use raw data but to store it in an altered, less sensitive form after its primary use. The drawbacks to this approach are similar to the drawbacks of not storing the data at all, except that now profile-based services are offered a trade off between the overhead of constantly requesting data and operating within a larger margin of uncertainty.

3.1.3. Data Access Policies

Our final type of privacy policy is the data access policy, which empowers users by allowing them to determine under what conditions a requesting entity is allowed to view or change a data item. As mentioned earlier, access is granted based on an agreement between the service or request specification and the data owner's privacy policy. One large benefit of data access policies is that they can eliminate many of the quality of service drawbacks that data collection and data storage policies incur. We can achieve this by creating an access storage policy that grants different views of data to different entities. That is, data can be *stored* one way and *viewed* differently by an entity (i.e. at a different precision and accuracy levels) based on the context of that entity's request. This would allow lower risk services to receive more sensitive data and higher risk services to receive less sensitive data but would require a middleware layer to manage to data views.

3.1.4. Notes on Data Collection and Storage Policies

We expect that some would argue that the idea of purposefully not collecting or storing data in a smart home system is impractical and imposes more problems than it solves. However, we emphasize that the purpose of a smart home is to make its inhabitants comfortable. When services or other data requestors specify their privacy policies, the privacy management system must trust 1) the validity of the specification and 2) that the specification will be upheld. If the service is intentionally or unintentionally misleading about its usage of data, the smart home has no way of detecting this abuse or enforcing the occupant's policy. Even if the abuse could be detected, as explained in [21], there is little legal precedent for handling such matters, and such precedents are not normally established quickly. Thus, with the absence of a trusted third party verifying service specifications and the lack of legal recourse for abused specifications, it may be more comfortable for smart home inhabitants to simply prevent certain types of data from being in the system.

3.2. On Realizing Context Inclusion

We argued earlier that privacy preferences are inherently contextual, depending on the situation in which a data request takes place and the person whose data is requested.

We now decompose the general notion of smart home context into data context, request context, occupant context, and environment context and briefly address how each relates to smart home privacy.

3.2.1. Data Context

We have already touched upon the issue of data context when we discussed data sensitivity. Recall that data sensitivity refers to the nature of the data, as well as its precision, accuracy, and freshness. These qualities also precisely capture our notion of data context. Occupants should be able to make policies that specify the sensitivities at which data enters, is used in, and leaves the system.

3.2.2. Request Context

We have also previously mentioned request context when discussing fair information practices. We recall that the factors affecting information practices are the purpose of the request, the actions to be taken on the data (including any subsequent release), the length of time the data is stored, how securely it is stored, and how secure the transmission of the data is. We add to this list the requested data's sensitivity, and the identity of requesting entity. Obviously, from this list we see that request contexts can become complicated very quickly and that some of these details may not need to be used for privacy policies. We will investigate these issues in further research.

3.2.3. Inhabitant Context

When considering the context of an inhabitant, or data owner, we note the existence of five general sub-contexts: location, activity, orientation (absolute or relative), emotion, and health. Of these, location, orientation, and health information seem to be the most privacy relevant. Although emotion detection research is still in its infancy, we posit it unlikely that many smart home occupants will want to define privacy policies based on their emotional state. Thus, inhabitants should be able to make privacy policies bases on where they are, what they are doing, and if it is an emergency or not.

3.2.4. Environment Context

Environment context represents the system state of the smart home. This includes such notions as time, security, safety, system load, network traffic, active and inactive service sets, and active and inactive device sets. However, many of these contexts will be of little concern to an occupant. Such low level environmental contexts as system load, service sets, and device sets are likely too fine-grained for occupants to be concerned with but are useful for security and other system administrative functions. We will investigate these issues in further research as well.

3.2.5. Context Concerns

Having identified the main components of smart home context, we now briefly address some issues associated with context management. One such issue in context-aware systems is how context should be represented. In current work, this is usually done using Role-Based Access Control (RBAC), logic predicates, or some combination of the two. [25] RBAC views context in terms of relationships, or roles, between entities, and associates access permissions with these roles. This approach has the benefit of reducing storage space as permissions are stored once per role as opposed to once per each entity assuming that role. However, the drawbacks of this approach include needing to decide which roles an entity can assume, when and how it can assume them, and making sure constraints among roles are upheld. Using logical predicates, on the other hand, has the advantage of not needing to maintain relationships between contexts but raises the issues of efficiently storing and dynamically evaluating contextual expressions.. In future work we plan on studying which representations are more suitable for which types of policies as well as which elements of each type of context are the most useful for privacy polices. We also note that whatever the internal context representation, we should avoid presenting inhabitants with too technical of an external representation because it could cause privacy management to become tedious and burdensome, leading to ineffective or inaccurate use.

3.3. On Realizing Non Intrusion

Again, non intrusion signifies limiting the number of unprompted communication exchanges with an inhabitant. Whether it be requesting consents or announcing services, the system should transparently handle as much as possible on the inhabitant's behalf. One particularly tricky application of this principle is privacy policy creation. In one approach, privacy policies could be created dynamically as the need for them arises. This would require the system to notify users when a new service is detected, provide a description of the new service to the inhabitant, and wait for a new privacy policy to be created before the service is activated. This will require a fair amount of manual effort from the user as each new service is added. Another possible approach would be to pre-define privacy policies before services are installed in the hopes that the policies will not need to be defined later. In contrast to the former technique, this would require more effort and careful planning at the outset of a smart home installation but less user interaction during system operation. Either way, both approaches require the existence of innovative policy management techniques as well as a simple and effective way of guiding users through policy creation. Policy management techniques will be addressed in future work, and the efficacy of any sort of user interface or training process falls under the realm of Human Computer Interaction (HCI) research.

Once the smart home system has obtained the privacy policies of its inhabitants, however that may be done, it should transparently control the comparison of privacy policies and request definitions, granting requests if and only no conflicts are found. For this to be accomplished, a machine readable policy specification must exist, as well as reliable and secure ways to retrieve and compare the policies. Some promising work in the area of privacy policy specification has been accomplished with P3P [3] and E-P3P [5], though both languages are not contextually expressive enough to support smart home context. Our future work will also look into extending such languages for use in smart homes.

4. Related Work

Generally speaking, existing privacy management efforts fall one of into two areas: those seeking to provide privacy of information gathered by public services or enterprises and those seeking to provide privacy of information requested from family members, peers, or co-workers. Whichever the case, no existing research effort combines all of the necessary types of context that affect a user's privacy within a smart home.

Research efforts that fall into the first category, like IBM's Enterprise Privacy Architecture [40], Langheinrich's Privacy Awareness System [20], He's Privacy-Aware Role-Based Access Control approach [17], the Usage Control model of Park et al. [24], and Fischer-Hübner's task-based privacy model [15], all use some type of request context, usually purpose specification or use limitation, to restrict data access. This is a necessary characteristic for smart home privacy management; however, these systems do not incorporate robust notions of environment or data owner contexts into their data access policies. Thus, they cannot fully provide the types of privacy policies required in smart homes.

Research efforts that fall into the second category, like InfoPriv [12, 13, 14], Context Fabric [19], and the efforts of Lederer et al. [22], do not use a common technique and therefore need to be addressed separately. The InfoPriv privacy model constructs information flow graphs based on privacy policies. In this system, information is only allowed to flow from one entity to another if there is a corresponding path in the system's information flow graph. This is a useful model to analyze and prevent violations resulting from the flow of information within an organization, but it is not applicable when considering third party systems. Also, this model is policy independent and therefore does not address any context surrounding data accesses. Context Fabric, on the other hand, focuses on the data owner, allowing him/her to create physical, social, or activity boundaries called information spaces. Permissions are associated with data objects in a particular set of information spaces, and violations occur when there is an unauthorized access within an information space or a data object crosses a boundary to an unauthorized space. This is a very innovative data owner-centric privacy model, but it also does not consider data accesses made by a third party system. The work of Lederer and company in [22], briefly mentioned earlier, focuses on providing different sensitivity levels of data to different entities. Allowing differences in data sensitivity is an important concept for maintaining privacy, but this work does not take into account the transfer of information between entities or notions such as request, environment, or occupant context during data access.

5. Conclusions and Future Work

In this work, we have identified and discussed many privacy issues in smart homes and defined principles to follow when designing a smart home privacy management system. These are Total Control, Equal Opportunity, Context Inclusion, and Non-Intrusion. We then discussed the implications of these principles and proposed the concepts of data collection, data storage, and data access policies. We also identified several areas for future research and elaborated on how existing privacy management schemes only partially fulfill privacy needs in smart homes due to a lack of contextual expression. Our future efforts will combine the approaches of existing works to provide more comprehensive privacy management in smart homes. We plan to do this by first formalizing our notions of privacy, context, and policy and then developing a prototype architecture for our system.

References

[1] European Commission. Directive 95/46/ec of the european parliament and of the council of 24 october 1995 on the protection of individuals with regard to the processing of personal data and on the free movement of such data, November 1995.

[2] Organization for Economic Co-operation and Development (OECD). Recommendation of the council concerning guidelines governing the protection of privacy and transborder flows of personal data, September 1980.

[3] W3C. Platform for Privacy Preferences. Available at www.w3.org/P3P.

[4] Angulo, C. and Tellez, R. Distributed Intelligence for Smart Home Applicances. In: Proceedings of the 16th International Joint Conference on Artificial. Intelligence, Denver CO, Morgan Kaufmann (1999) pp. 1356–1361.

[5] Ashley, P., Hada, S., Karjoth, G., and Schunter, M. In: Proceedings of the ACM Workshop on Privacy in the Electronic Society (WPES), 2002.

[6] Beckwith, R. Designing for Ubiquity: The Perception of Privacy. In: IEEE Pervasive Computing, vol. 2. pp 40-46, April-June 2003.

[7] Blaine, A. Price, Karim A, and Bashar, N. Keeping Ubiquitous Computing to Yourself: A practical model for user control of privacy.

[8] Cas, J. Privacy in Pervasive Computing Environments. A Contradiction in Terms. In: IEEE Technology and Society Magazine, Spring 2005, pp. 24-33.

[9] Cook, D., Huber, M. Gopalratnam, K., and Youngblood, M. (2003) Learning to Control a Smart Home Environment.

[10] Convington, M., Long W., Srinivasan, S., Dey, A, Ahamad, M., and Abowd, G. Securing Context-Aware Applications Using Environment Roles. (2001) College of Computing. Georgia Institute of Technology, Atlanta, GA. Available: http://www.cc.gatech.edu/fce/ctk/pubs/SACMAT2001.pdf

[11] Dey, A. Abowd, G., and Salber, D. (1999) A Context Based Infrastructure for Smart Environments.

[12] Dreyer, L. and Olivier, M. A Workbench for Privacy Policies, Proc. of 22ndAnnual International Computer Software and Applications Conference (COMPSAC'98), pp. 350-355, IEEE, 1998.

[13] Dreyer, L. and Olivier, M. Dynamic Aspects of the InfoPriv Model for Information Privacy, Proc. of the 9th International Workshop on Database and Expert Systems Applications, pp. 340-345, IEEE, 1998.

[14] Dreyer, L. and Olivier, M. An Information-Flow Model for Privacy (InfoPriv). In S Jajodia (editor), Database Security XII: Status and Prospects, pp. 77-90, Kluwer, 1999.

[15] Fischer-Hübner, S. IT-Security and Privacy, Lecture Notes in Computer Science 1958 (LNCS 1958), Springer-Verlag, 2001.

[16] Ghorbel, M., Segarra M., Kerdreux J., Keryell R., Thepaut A., and Mokhtar, M. Networking and Communication in Smart Home for People with Disabilities. Proc. of the 9th International Conference on Computers Helping People (ICCHP), 2004.

[17] He, Q. Privacy Enforcement with an Extended Role-Based Access Control Model. NCSU Computer Science Technical Report. 2003

[18] Karjoth, G., Schunter, M., Waidner, M. Privacy-enabled Services for Enterprises. Proc.of the 13th International Workshop on Database and Expert Systems Applications (DEXA'02), IEEE, 2002

[19] Jiang, X. and Landay, J. Modeling Privacy Control in Context-Aware Systems, IEEE Pervasive Computing, Volume 1 Issue 3, pp. 59-63, July-September, 2002.

[20] Langheinrich, M. A Privacy Awareness System for Ubiquitous Computing Environments. In: Proc. of the 4th International Conference on Ubiquitous Computing (UbiComp 2002), Sep. 2002.

[21] Langheinrich, M."Privacy by Design—Principles of Privacy-Aware Ubiquitous Systems," Proc. 3rd Int'l Conf. Ubiquitous Computing, Springer-Verlag, 2001, pp. 273–291.

[22] Lederer, S., Hong, J. Jiang, X., Dey, A. Landay, J. and Manko, J.: 2003, `Towards Everyday Privacy for Ubiquitous Computing'. Technical Report UCB-CSD-03-1283, Computer Science Division, University of California, Berkeley.

[23] Meye S. and Rakotonirainy. A. A Survey of Research on Context-Aware Homes. In: Workshop on Wearable, Invisible, Context-Aware, Ambient, Pervasive and Ubiquitous Computing, Adelaide, Australia. Conferences in Research and Practice in Information Technology, Vol. 21.

[24] Park, J. and Sandhu, R. Towards Usage Control Models: Beyond Traditional Access Control, Proc. of the 7th ACM Symposium on Access Control Models and Technologies (SACMAT'02), Monterey, CA, pp. 57-64, ACM, 2002

[25] Sandhu, R., Coyne, E., Feinstein, H., and Youman, C. Role-Based Access Control Models, In: IEEE Computer, Volume 29 Issue 2, pp. 38–47, Feb. 1996.

Promoting Independence for Older Persons with Disabilities
W.C. Mann and A. Helal (Eds.)
IOS Press, 2006

Integrating Intelligent Systems for Elder Care in RoboCare

Amedeo CESTA [a,1], and Federico PECORA [a,b]
[a] *Institute for Cognitive Science and Technology, Italian National Research Council, Rome, Italy*
[b] *Department of Systems and Informatics (DIS) of the University of Rome, Rome, Italy*

Abstract. This article describes the highlights of the first two years of activities of RoboCare, an Italian research project aimed at developing intelligent software and robotic agents which can enhance the quality of life of elderly people at home or in a health-care institution. These two years of research have produced several innovations related to the use of robotics, sensory, and activity monitoring technology in the elder-care context. This paper provides a summary of the main contributions of RoboCare in its first two years of activities. Rather than describing in detail the specific techniques we have developed, for which we point the interested reader to related work, our aim is to highlight some specific issues which our results have given rise to in the context of AI applications in elder care. More specifically, the paper is dedicated to exposing the principal strengths and weaknesses of our technology in this application scenario.

Keywords. Intelligent systems, robotics, elder care, assistive technology

1. Introduction

This article describes the highlights of the first two years of activities of RoboCare, an Italian research project aimed at developing and studying the applicability of AI techniques for the care of the elderly. The RoboCare project focuses on the development of distributed systems in which software and robotic agents contribute to the common goal of generating active services in environments in which humans may need assistance and guidance. In particular, we are pursuing the idea of developing support technology which can play a role in allowing vulnerable elderly people to lead an independent lifestyle in their own homes.

Recent statistics show how the population in Europe is slowly getting older. Increasing attention has therefore been given to the issue of "independence" and "aging at home", and support tools have been developed to ensure that elderly and partially impaired people can continue to enjoy an independent lifestyle. For this reason, since its beginning research in RoboCare has followed two tracks by focusing on the following scenarios:

1.1. Domestic environment

The RoboCare Domestic Environment (RDE – see Figure 1) is an experimental setup which recreates a three-room flat. It is intended as a testbed environment in which to test the ability of the domotic technology built by the various research units, such as non-intrusive monitoring, domestic robots and environmental supervision.

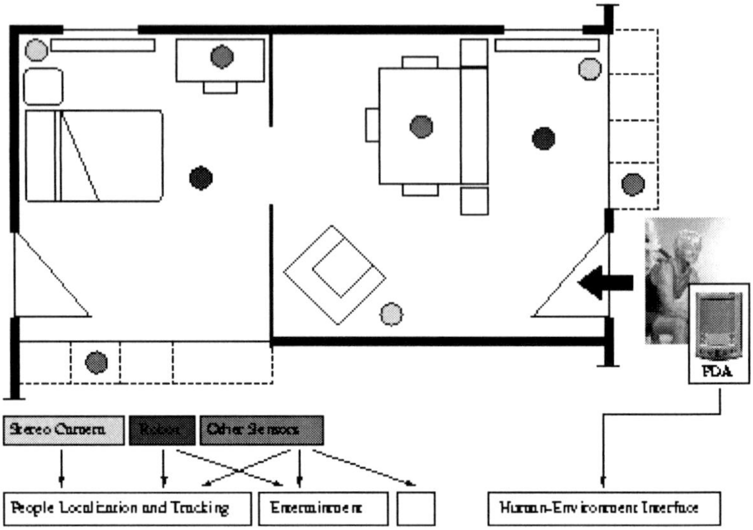

Figure 1 Three-room flat mock-up of an elderly person's domestic environment.

1.2. Health-care institution

The health-care scenario focuses on analyzing the possible deployment of an array of software and robotic components to facilitate complex workflows which require the coordination of human personnel and artificial agents in the context of a large institution (see Figure 2). The role of an intelligent supervisor in this scenario is to synthesize and monitor the current execution of complex plans which involve the use of heavy-duty robotic platforms, capable of moving in large spaces, walking or transporting people, as well as performing environmental supervisory tasks. Various research units operate in this scenario by means of simulations, while others contribute by developing large robots, which are more suitable for this environment.

RoboCare mainly focuses on the following four fields of research: *robotic platforms*, *sensory systems*, *activity supervision in complex environments*, and *human-technology interaction*. Rather than describing in detail the specific techniques we have developed, for which we point the interested reader to related work, we dedicate the following paragraphs to (1) a brief overview of the main results obtained in these first two years of activities in these four fields of research, and (2) a discussion on some lessons learned and an outlook to future developments which have emerged in the process of our attempts to customize AI technology for elder care.

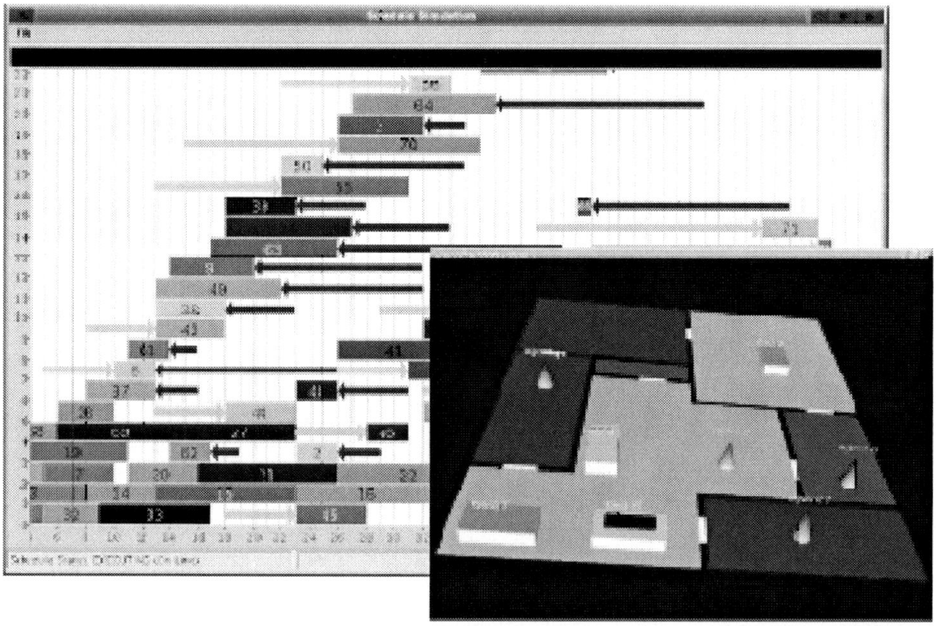

Figure 2 Task supervision system at work on a floor of the simulated health-care institution environment.

2. Main Research Tracks

It is important to emphasize that the main objective of RoboCare is to investigate the integration of robotic, sensory and automated reasoning components into the domestic and health-care institution scenarios. In this sense, the target application does not consist primarily in the development of the single components, rather in a single service-providing support infrastructure for elder care in a domestic or health-care institution context. Also, RoboCare does not focus primarily on robotics. Nonetheless, robotics has an important role because of its contribution to two demos aimed at showcasing our results at the end of the third year (RDE and institution environments). This objective is being pursued in a bottom-up fashion: the first year of activities has focused on singling out and developing the basic functionalities of the single components, such as the people localization and tracking sensory system, the basic robotic capabilities and the symbolic reasoning modules for the supervisory agents. Starting from these basic functionalities, the second year of the project has focused on integration in the two scenarios.

Research in RoboCare deals with two main aspects related to technology for elderly care: on one hand, the development of the enabling domotic components for deployment in the target scenarios (such as intelligent sensors and robotic platforms), and on the other the development of the service-providing software infrastructure which makes use of the functionalities provided by the domotic components (such as activity supervision and diagnostics). Clearly, the implementation of this technology within the specific applicative context of RoboCare has lead to extensive investigation in the areas of human-computer and human-robot interaction, with two distinct research units dealing exclusively with these topics. More in particular, the principal research areas and results are summarized below, along with references which the interested reader can follow for more in-depth analyses on specific topics.

2.1. Robotic platforms

One of the most fundamental abilities a mobile robot must have in order to carry out even the simplest task in the environment is that of being capable of deducing its current position in the environment. This problem is known in the literature as *localization*. A large body of research has been dedicated to this problem, as detailed in [12,13], in which various approaches are studied, such as SLAM (simultaneous localization and mapping) through laser-range finders and Kalman filters.

Along with localization, another important issue which is being addressed is *safe navigation*, which consists in the ability of a mobile robot (such as robotic wheelchairs) to plan trajectories which involve smooth curves and maximize the distance from obstacles [7,16].

Mobile robots have also been equipped with basic *people following* capabilities, as reported in [10], as well as some *manipulatory* skills by means of a robotic arm which can be programmed by example [1].

Overall, the robotic functionalities which have been implemented during the first year thus allow robust and safe robot navigation in domestic and health-care institution environments, and basically consist in the "go-to-position", "follow-person" and "follow-robot" behaviors. These functionalities have been integrated on both small robots for domestic use (e.g., ActiveMedia Pioneer equipped with touch-screen and tray) and on a heavy-duty robot named Staffetta developed at the University of Genoa, which is used in the larger institution scenario (see Figure 3).

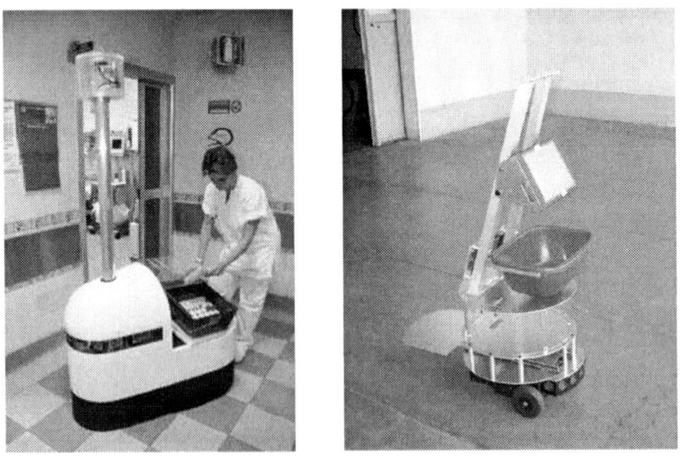

Figure 3 The Staffetta robot used in the HCI scenario (left), and the modified ActiveMedia Pioneer robot for the RDE (right).

2.2. Sensory systems

Sensors are a particularly important part of the development process, as they provide a bridge between the physical world of the target scenario and the high level reasoning capabilities of the supervision agents, which rely on a symbolic representation of the real world. Sensors must be intelligent in that they must interpret raw data and build from it this symbolic layer. Moreover, this process is subject to strong real-time constraints.

One of the first basic services to have been developed consists in *people/robot localization and tracking*. This sensor consists of a stereo-camera and a series of image processing algorithms aimed at singling out and tracking multiple persons (or robots) in 3D space [2]. Along with these tracking capabilities, which provide *gesture/posture recognition* sensors [6] have been developed with the aim of providing a visual means of communication between the intelligent environment and an assisted elderly person. Thus, the vision-based environmental sensors implement functionalities such as "where-is-person/robot" queries, as well as basic human- robot/computer/intelligent environment communication by means of body posture and hand movement recognition.

Furthermore, various *human feature recognition* techniques have been studied, such as facial recognition systems based on hybrid feature-invariant/SVM methods [8], as well as other biometric techniques for person recognition [9].

2.3. Activity supervision in complex environments

Whether in the domestic care or health care institution scenario, one of the most important aspects of the prototypes we are trying to achieve is the ability to reconstruct the state of the environment and of the assisted person(s) through the symbolic representations provided by the sensors. To this end, our research has focused on three issues.

First, work by the University of Turin [14] has developed a platform for *multi-agent system diagnostics* in the context of a health-care institution scenario. Given a complex schedule of activities to be performed by a multitude of robotic agents in a large institution, and given the fact that most of the agents' tasks are highly interdependent, the ability to diagnose the state of the system is fundamental for correct plan execution and contingency reaction. This task is carried out by the diagnostics module, which is capable of integrating the (partial) information on the state of the agents and of the tasks they are carrying out in order to quickly infer possible execution-time failures and their causes.

Alongside the diagnostics capabilities, the ISTC-CNR research unit is attempting to provide a proactive functionality, namely a complete *caregiver console for non-intrusive supervision*. The aim is twofold: first, to develop a software supervisor which is capable of monitoring the adherence of the daily activities of an assisted elderly person in the RDE to a set of predefined behavioral constraints [4]; second, to orchestrate the available domotic services (robots, intelligent household appliances, etc.) according to the requirements of the assisted person, a task which can be cast as a planning problem [15]. This real-time execution monitoring relies on a CSP representation of what we call a "behavioral pattern", which represents a collection of complex time constraints on certain activities the assisted person may carry out during the day. These constraints in turn represent the inter-dependencies between daily tasks a caregiver may want to enforce; the violation of each constraint can be independently associated to a different reaction strategy, which can go from simple log registration or alarms which trigger the intervention of a human being, to the on-line generation of complex reaction schemes which involve the caregivers and the software/robotic agents.

In addition, a distinct research unit is investigating the issue of *safe planning* by means of QBF (quantified boolean formula) verification [5], where the underlying idea is to cast a planning problem along with a set of safety constraints into a problem which can be solved by means of an efficient QBF solver.

2.4. Interaction between humans and technological artifacts

The numerous issued related to the acceptance of the technology developed by RoboCare are being addressed by two distinct research units. On one hand, some work has investigated and provided a taxonomy of different modalities of *human-robot interaction*, as reported in [3], particularly focusing on human-robot communication.

As for technology acceptance, the ISTC's Environmental Psychology unit has begun an investigation into *lay-peoples' attitudes towards technology* [11,17]. The particular focus of this work is to explore the expectations of targeted groups of elderly people towards the potential benefits of robotics and domotics in general, such as safety, comfort, etc. An in-depth study was conducted on the dependency of their inclinations on age-group, education, and other influential factors. This analysis has revealed that a large category of elderly persons (particularly those below the age of 75) are rather favorable to embedding technological components into their homes.

3. AI Technology in Elder Care

Overall, RoboCare represents an effort to understand what sort of support tools can be obtained by integrating today's state-of-the-art AI technology in an off-the-shelf manner. The challenge is to assess the extent to which the above mentioned techniques can provide a cost-effective means for building these off-the-shelf components for assistive technology. The following section attempts to sketch an outlook based on the results obtained after the second year of activities.

The following considerations are organized in three parts. First, we consider the issues related to the use of robotic platforms for elder care. We then comment on the adequacy of the sensory capabilities we have achieved, and we finally focus on the added value of AI reasoning technology for non-intrusive supervision.

3.1. Robotic Platforms

The state-of-the-art in robotic platforms has allowed us to develop mobile robots with robust navigation capabilities. Through the use of different techniques, we have successfully deployed these platforms in both the domestic and the health-care institution scenarios. Yet one critical question still remains to be answered: what sort of meaningful support functionalities can mobile robots effectively provide for domestic use by an elderly person or in the context of a large health-care institution? Indeed, one of the principal aims of RoboCare is to provide an answer to this question.

So far, one interesting conclusion we can draw from our two-year experience is that we have ascertained that there is still a great deal of work to be done in order to effectively employ robots for elderly care. The first two years of this project have primarily focused on the development of robust localization, mapping and navigation techniques. While the results obtained are important and in line with the state-of-the-art in robotics research, they also mirror the large gap between state-of-the-art and application of robotic technology for elder care. The principal reason for this gap lies in the lack of off-the-shelf components providing functionalities which are advanced enough for deployment. While it is clearly possible to produce highly specialized robotic platforms for caretaking purposes, it is also clear that this sort of technology also comes at a very high price in terms of both hardware and software development. For the general-purpose robots we have employed in RoboCare, it is necessary to further invest in the high-end capabilities, by means for instance of specific projects aimed at developing manipulatory add-ons as well as other high level cognitive capabilities. This would certainly contribute to increasing the availability of complex and commercially-viable robotic platforms which could be applied more directly in the context of elder care.

Nonetheless, there are a number of very good reasons to invest in robots for the care of the elderly. One of them lies in the expectations elderly people have of robots. Recent surveys (e.g., [11]) have shown these to be very compelling arguments for having an assistive robot at home, yet quite out of reach for today's off-the-shelf robotic platform. Another compelling reason is related to embodiment. This is a characteristic in which elderly people are particularly interested in, expressing preferences such as "it should look like a child" or "it should not frighten the cat". Meeting these requirements while affording the functionalities elderly people would like in a robot is a big challenge for roboticists, and will lead to interesting developments in the future.

3.2. Sensory capabilities

The RoboCare project has largely focused on artificial vision technology for people/robot localization and tracking, as well as person, posture and gesture recognition. High-performance CPUs and video processors, as well as relatively cheap medium-range cameras available today have allowed us to develop algorithms for achieving complex artificial vision functionalities. The step to bundling this software in self-contained and easily deployable "intelligent sensors" is well in reach. Currently available technology is capable of providing services such as people tracking and recognition, as well as interpreting gestures and diagnosing the state of a person based on posture.

Overall, we envisage that we will soon be able to count on a large amount of information from static artificial vision sensors deployed within the environment. This information can be used to provide services which may indeed be of use in an elderly person's home. For instance, a "lost and found" functionality could be set up relatively simply: a central supervisor maintains a database of all non-static objects within the field of view of the cameras, e.g., glasses, keys, hat, scarf, etc. Upon request, the system can be summoned to provide answers to queries such as "what have I done with my glasses?" Perhaps even more interestingly, the system may be programmed to start by providing only "hints" in order to point the assisted person to the lost object, a feature which is attractive for mildly-affected Alzheimer patients.

In conclusion, our two years of experience with RoboCare have allowed us to develop a series of specific artificial vision techniques which can be employed with commonly available hardware components in order to provide interesting services for the care of the elderly, and which are also relatively close to being readily deployable.

3.3. Non-Intrusive Supervision

Given the focus on integration, one of the primary aims of RoboCare is to develop a software infrastructure which can serve as an interface between human caregivers or the assisted elderly persons and the intelligent environment as a whole. This overall "controller" is composed of a variety of different planning, scheduling, and constraint reasoning algorithms, all of which provide the representation and reasoning capabilities for activity supervision, diagnosis, and execution monitoring. The integration effort has focused on making these many functionalities accessible in the form of a "caregiver console", a group of interfaces which subsume the technology-related aspects of the underlying representations and provide a highly customized control panel for supervising and configuring the overall behavior of the intelligent home.

One important issue we are beginning to address now is related to information integration. More precisely, the amount and complexity of the symbolic information we can obtain from the sensory subsystem (in order of difficulty: objects, people, complex situations, ... – see sensory capabilities above) is steadily increasing. We envisage that we will soon be able to count on a large amount of high-level information form the intelligent sensors. This forebodes the development of more elaborate reasoning capabilities, which in turn will allow to increase the effectiveness of the intelligent environment in real every-day situations. At this point of development we are capable of implementing a rather stable sensor-supervisor loop which allows to track some key behaviors of the assisted elderly person in his or her daily routines. Yet while the state of the art reasoners which are being employed are for now sufficiently powerful and well-suited for dealing with the combinatorial problems of the RDE, it is possible that as the sensors grow in complexity we will have to extend their capabilities in order to accommodate more elaborate forms of reasoning. In particular, the current solvers are direct relatives of research prototypes, and as such are not "tuned" for use in this particular applicative context. One of the main efforts which will have to be made will probably consist in enhancing the expressiveness of the automated reasoning tools in order to accommodate requirements which are more suitable for the elder care context.

Another interesting issue which is beginning to emerge and which has not been fully addressed yet is the acceptance of automated supervision. On one hand, an automated supervisor can be configured to share only a small part of the information with humans, extracting from the detailed logs of the assisted person's activities only the aggregated information which is meaningful from the point of view of the caregiver. Our hypothesis, which still needs to be validated by an in-depth analysis, is that 24/7 monitoring by means of fixed environmental sensors can be acceptable as long as the data is processed by computers and only a subset of previously agreed upon results are then submitted to human caregivers – notice that this hypothesis underlies the acceptance of targeted advertisement mechanisms, such as some email clients which automatically parse your email and provide advertisement links which are related to the parsed text. Obviously, only a detailed analysis can assess in which types of situations this approach is acceptable, yet we believe that it may be indeed feasible if this "habit-tracking" technology can contribute to a prolonged independent lifestyle.

Acknowledgments

This research is partially supported by MIUR (Italian Ministry of Education, University and Research) under project RoboCare: "A Multi-Agent System with Intelligent Fixed and Mobile Robotic Components", L. 449/97 (http://robocare.istc.cnr.it).

References

[1] J. Aleotti, S. Caselli, and G. Maccherozzi. "Trajectory reconstruction with nurbs curves for robot programming by demonstration". In *IEEE International Conference on Computational Intelligence in Robotics and Automation, CIRA, 2005.*

[2] S. Bahadori, L. Iocchi, G.R. Leone, D. Nardi, and L. Scozzafava. "Real-Time People Localization and Tracking throught Fized Stereo Vision". In *Proceedings of Industrial and Engineering Applications of Artificial Intelligence and Expert Systems (IEA/AIE), 2005.*

[3] A. Cappelli, E. Giovannetti, and M. Federico. "The Role of Communication in Human-Robot Interaction". In *Proceedings of the Second Robocare Workshop, ISTC-CNR, Rome (Italy), 2005.*

[4] A. Cesta, G. Cortellessa, F. Pecora, and R. Rasconi. "Monitoring Domestic Activities with Scheduling Techniques". In *Proceedings of the Second Robocare Workshop, ISTC-CNR, Rome (Italy), 2005.*

[5] M. De Luca, E. Giunchiglia, M. Narizzano, and A. Tacchella. "Safe Planning as a QBF evaluation problem". In *Proceedings of the Second Robocare Workshop, ISTC-CNR, Rome (Italy), 2005.*

[6] H. Dindo, A. Chella, and I Infantino. "A System for simultaneous People Tracking and Posture Recognition in the context of Human-Robot Interaction". In *Proceedings of the Second Robocare Workshop, ISTC-CNR, Rome (Italy), 2005.*

[7] A. Farinelli, L. Iocchi, and D. Nardi. "Path Planning in a Domestic Dynamic Environment". In *Proceedings of the First Robocare Workshop, ISTC-CNR, Rome (Italy), 2003.*

[8] S. Ferrari, I. Frosio, V. Piuri, and N.A. Borghese. "Automatic multi-scale meshing through HRBF Networks". In *IEEE Trans. Instrumentation & Measurement, 2005.*

[9] M. Gamassi, V. Piuri, D. Sana, and F. Scotti. "Robust fingerprint detection for access control". In *Proceedings of the Second Robocare Workshop, ISTCCNR, Rome (Italy), 2005.*

[10] O. Gigliotta, M. Caretti, S. Shokur, and S. Nolfi. "Toward a Person-Follower Robot". In *Proceedings of the Second Robocare Workshop, ISTC-CNR, Rome (Italy), 2005.*

[11] M.V. Giuliani, M. Scopelliti, and F. Fornara. "Coping strategies and technology in later life". In *Proceedings of AISB 2005 - Symposium Robot Companions: Hard Problems and Open Challenges in Robot-Human Interaction , Hatfield, UK, 2005.*

[12] G. Grisetti, C. Stachniss, andW. Burgard. "Improving grid-based SLAM with rao-blackwellized particle filters by adaptive proposals and selective resampling". In *Proceedings of the IEEE International Conference on Robotics and Automation (ICRA 05), 2005.*

[13] F. Mastrogiovanni, A. Sgorbissa, and R. Zaccaria. "On The Tips of One s Toes: Self-localization in a Dynamic Environment". In *IEEE International Conference on Computational Intelligence in Robotics and Automation, CIRA, 2005.*

[14] R. Micalizio, P. Torasso, and G. Torta. "On-Line Monitoring and Diagnosis of Multi-Agent Systems: a Model Based Approach". In *Proceedings of ECAI, Valencia, Spain, pages 848 852, 2004.*

[15] F. Pecora and A. Cesta. "Evaluating Plans through Restrictiveness and Resource Strength". In *Proceedings of the 2nd Workshop on Integrating Planning into Scheduling (WIPIS) at AAAI-05, Pittsburgh, USA, 2005.*

[16] A. Scalzo and G. Veruggio. "People following and guiding with a nonholonomic slow steering robot". In *Proceedings of the First RoboCare Workshop, ISTC-CNR, Rome (Italy), 2005.*

[17] M. Scopelliti and M.V. Giuliani. "If I had a robot at home... People's representation of domestic robots". In *S. Keates, J. Clarkson, P. Langdon, and P. Robinson, editors, Design for a more inclusive world, pages 257 266. Springer Verlag, 2004.*

Promoting Independence for Older Persons with Disabilities
W.C. Mann and A. Helal (Eds.)
IOS Press, 2006

Steward Robot for Human-Friendly Assistive Home Environment

Z. Zenn BIEN [a,1], Hyong-Euk LEE[a], Young-Min KIM[b], Yong-Hwi KIM[a], Jin-Woo JUNG[b] and Kwang-Hyun PARK[a]
[a]*Department of Electrical Engineering and Computer Science, KAIST, Yuseong-Gu, Daejeon, KOREA*
[b]*Human-friendly Welfare Robot System Research Center, KAIST, Yuseong-Gu, Daejeon, KOREA*

Abstract. In this paper, we propose a steward robot system in the human-friendly assistive home environment for the independent living of persons who are elderly or disabled. In the view of extended concept of services robot, steward robot becomes an efficient intermediate agent between the potential user and the complex control environment with its learning and emotional interaction capability. Two different types (software type and hardware type) of steward robots are introduced which have been developed in the Intelligent Sweet Home (KAIST).

Introduction

Promoting independence for older people and people with disabilities in their living environment becomes an imperative notion for all societies in the years to come. As an approach to achieve "independence", this paper addresses the problem of controlling an assistive home environment emphasizing a human-friendly man-machine interaction. From the functional point of view, a house is gradually shifting from a basic shelter toward a large-scale system including various assistive subsystems playing their inherent roles to provide the residents with comfortable living conditions, independence and quality of life. However, the increase of the number and complexity of subsystems, to enhance available services in a smart home, could lead to a decrease of convenience, accessibility and cost effectiveness, since it is difficult to control all the services using many corresponding HMIs (Human-Machine Interfaces). The mode of interaction between the resident and the subsystems is thus a significant aspect in the design of a smart home especially for older persons and people with disabilities.

Therefore, we propose the concept of 'steward robot', which can help or guide the inhabitant to operate all the above-explained subsystems easily in a smart home environment. Literally, steward means one employed in a large household or estate to manage domestic concerns such as supervision of servants, collection of rents, and keeping of accounts. We apply this meaning to the robotic agent in the intelligent house to perform the role of steward for the inhabitant. That is, steward robot can be an intermediate agent between the complex smart house system and the end-user to enhance usability and convenience.

In this paper, steward robot, called Joseph, is introduced as a part of Intelligent Sweet Home(ISH)[1]. There are two types of Joseph: 1) software type robot virtual

Joseph, 2) hardware type robot Joseph. Virtual Joseph is composed of its virtual 3D avatar and its intelligent processing module with learning and emotional interaction capability. Hardware type robot Joseph is now in development, to provide pro-active services and perform human-friendly interaction tasks including the function of virtual Joseph's.

1. Intelligent Sweet Home(ISH) and Steward Robot

ISH is a service robot-integrated intelligent house platform with a sensor-based home network system, which provides various kinds of daily living assistive tasks for the inhabitant (e.g. serving a meal/drink, assisting walk, delivering a newspaper, etc.). In particular, it is designed for people with serious difficulties in doing daily tasks. Assistive devices or systems such as ISH will be very helpful in assisting people thereby providing as much independence as possible, and improving their quality of life.

Our work is distinguished in the sense of fully supporting indispensable daily tasks with various functionalities to comply with the needs of the users from the statistical and questionnaire survey [2], and is based on the idea that the technologies and solutions for such a smart house should be human-friendly, i.e. smart houses should possess a high level of intelligence in their control, actions and interactions with the users, offering them high level of comfort and functionality. The effectiveness of smart houses for its inhabitants is strongly dependent on the devices in the home environment and the efficiency of the automatic system that synchronizes their operation. The mode of interaction of the inhabitant with the home-installed devices is also a significant aspect of the smart house design. As a solution, Intelligent Sweet Home consists of several assistive systems and human-friendly interfaces (Fig. 1)

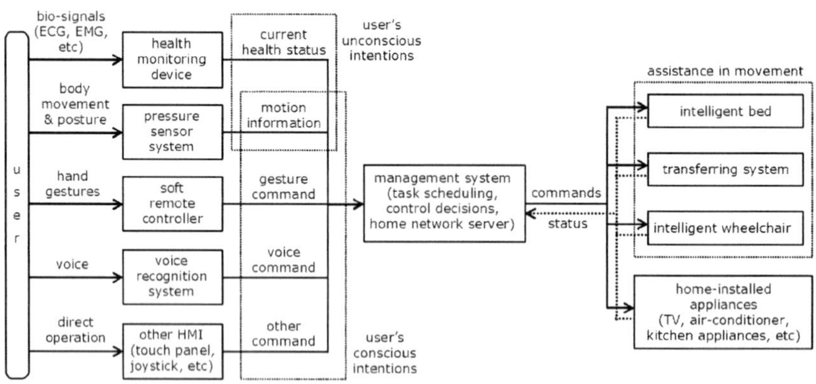

Figure 1. Block diagram of ISH

These assistive systems provide many of services for the inhabitant. However, its complex control interfaces may be an inconvenience. To reduce this inconvenience, the steward robot can be an effective unified human-machine interface, acting as the *manager*.

For example, if the person with spinal cord injury wants to go outside from the bed, he has to do the following sequence in ISH: 1) Control the lifting system to transfer him/herself to the wheelchair, 2) Control the wheelchair system at the appropriate position for docking the lift system, 3) let the lift system go on the recharging place, 4) let all the home appliance shut down, 5) let ISH be on the security mode. In this case, the user has to control each device with proper sequence. But if a certain robot agent can learn these complex sequences, it can schedule/manage the tasks of each device with a single command. In this way, steward robot can be a manager robot in the home environment.

Another issue is its *interaction capability*. With conventional service robots, the robotic agent's role is a simple slave machine. That is, the robot agent executes given orders by the owner without any interaction. However, we propose the concept of a steward, as an enhanced service robot with interaction capability. This robot requires the following functions: 1) provide personalized services in advance of the owner's command using intention reading techniques with learning capability, and reflecting the owner's satisfaction degree on the knowledge database of living behavior pattern, 2) is a human-friendly interactive agent with its own emotional expression. In this sense, learning and emotional interaction capabilities are essential components in the proposed concept of steward robot.

Additionally, this software type robot has merit in the sense of accessibility. Through the wired/wireless communication network, the user can access the steward robot everywhere using personal computing interfaces (e.g. PCs, PDA, cellular phone). The hardware type robot can increase the quality as well as the quality of services. If the robot agent has a manipulator and mobile platform, it can provide pro-active services for the inhabitant (e.g. delivering a meal, pick up an object below).

The software type virtual Joseph has been implemented with learning and emotional interaction capability. The hardware type Joseph is now being developed with the functions of virtual Joseph's.

2. Virtual Steward Robot

2.1. Structure of virtual steward robot

The block diagram of virtual Joseph and ISH components are shown in the Figure 2. Commands from the inhabitant by various HMIs and the status information from health/environmental monitoring /sensing devices are collected in the home-network server. Virtual Joseph has authority to access the home-network server. The inhabitant can access subsystems in ISH directly using HMIs, and can use virtual Joseph to control subsystems indirectly with voice commands.

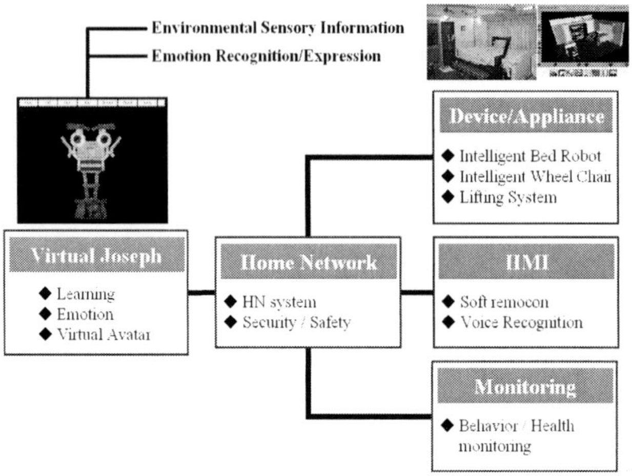

Figure 2. Block diagram of virtual Joseph and ISH

Figure 3 shows the internal structure of virtual Joseph. Learning capability enables machines/robots to understand humans and provides personalized services depending on the user's preferences and his/her living behavior pattern. By collecting environmental sensory information and inhabitant's command history to the target subsystem such as robotic agents and home-network system, the learning system could reveal the empirical patterns from incrementally drawn set of behaviors, and attempt to appropriately control the target devices through intention reading. For more human-friendly interaction between a human and a robot, virtual Joseph generates and expresses its own emotional state to the inhabitant through a 3D avatar model.

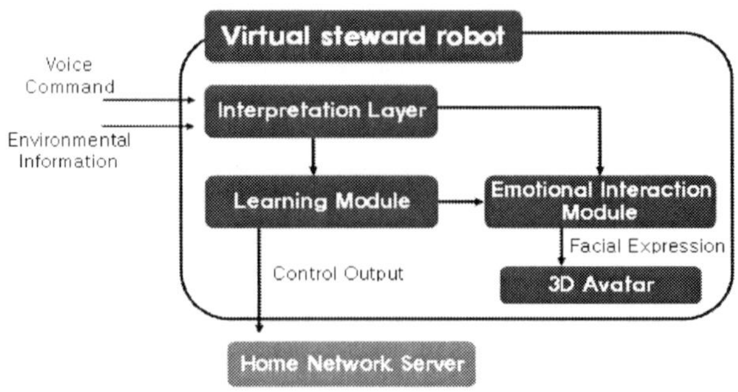

Figure 3. Internal structure of virtual steward robot

2.2. *Emotional Interaction Capability: Facial Expression Generation*

The EI (emotional interaction) system of virtual steward robot is basically based on OCC[6] emotion model from psychology. In psychology, there are two major branches of human emotion modeling, which can be applied for the emotion generation system of the robot system. Table 1 shows characteristics and merits/demerits of these two models.

Because of its geometrical representation, the dimensional model is an easy to understand mapping of the relation between emotion standards (dimensions) and the corresponding emotions. However, it can handle only basic emotions, and the physical meaning of its standards are too abstract to apply to the engineering system. That is, a system designer has difficulty in mapping potential input attributes (e.g. external stimulus, drives) to the corresponding standards.

On the other hand, the OCC model is based on interaction-related emotion words, which can be intuitively assigned from the observation of human interaction. Figure 4 describes an overall structure of the OCC emotion model. The tree-structured model has branches representing three main dimensions – consequences of an event, praiseworthiness of the agent, aspect of the object. At the end of the branches, two emotion words which have opposite meanings, are generated. Using this model, Otony[6][7] determined that 22 emotion words related to real interaction could be generated.

Table 1. Human's emotion models

		Dimensional model[3][4][5]	OCC model[6][7][8]
	A point of view	Characterizing emotion words	Origin of emotions
	Standards (Dimensions)	valence, arousal, stance, control, etc.	valence + event, agent, object
	Handling emotions	Basic emotions	22 complex emotions
Applying to sociable robot(agent)	Advantages	-Geometric representation of emotion space	-Intuitive meaning of dimension -Interaction-based complex emotion's representation
	Disadvantages	-Abstract meaning of dimension -Limitation of mapping complex emotions	- Limitation of representing the strength or intensity of an emotion
	Examples	KISMET Project[9], Humanoid cranium Project[10]	OZ Project[11]

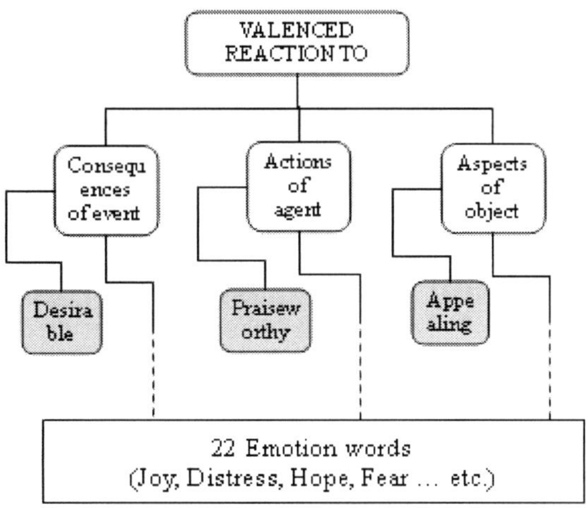

Figure 4. Overall structure of OCC model

However, Otony also concluded that it requires a complex system to apply this emotion model in real situations. Therefore, among 22 possible emotions, 8 emotions were selected for virtual steward robot regarding interaction scenarios between a steward robot and its owner: Joy/Distress, Pride/Shame, Hope/Fear, Like/Dislike. The selected emotional state is represented through facial expression of 3D avatar (Fig. 5).

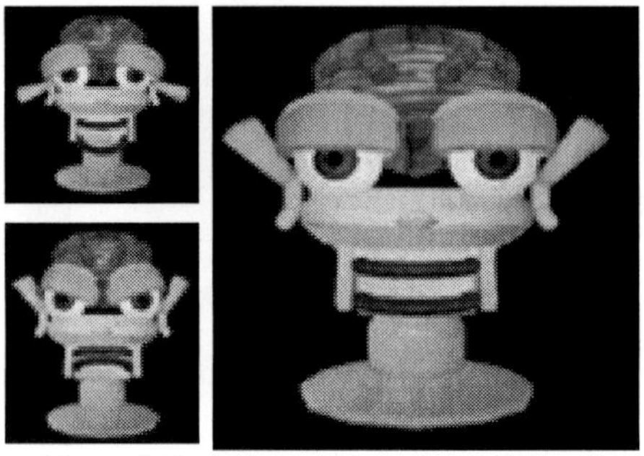

Figure 5. Facial Expression of virtual Joseph

2.3. *Learning Capability: Learning Living Behavior Pattern*

There are several application platforms of a smart home which deal with the living behavior pattern learning problem. Adaptive House (University of Colorado) [12] has been developed in the sense of an optimal heating/lighting control scheme to minimize energy and discomfort cost using environmental sensory information by ANN (Artificial Neural Network). iDorm (University of Essex) [13,14] controls various home appliances automatically based on the inhabitant's life style by fuzzy rule-based incremental learning technique. However, in both application systems, there is some limitation in the view of knowledge discovery.

By simple definition, KDD(Knowledge Discovery in Database) is the nontrivial process of identifying valid, novel, potentially useful, and ultimately understandable patterns in data[15]. ANN has been used widely in the pattern classification problem but it doesn't provide understandable knowledge because accumulated knowledge is expressed only in the numerical weight values between neurons. In this sense, fuzzy if-then rule type expression by FL (Fuzzy Logic) can be effective for knowledge discovery because FL can make knowledge database similar to the way humans think with its fuzzy term and association rules from uncertain data.

Therefore, KD(Knowledge Discovery) is redefined as extracting the consistent fuzzy if-then rule between input pattern and desired output in this paper. Also, it includes constructing an appropriate fuzzy partition for each input space for associating rules.

In this sense, the FL-based approach of iDorm is preferred over the one used in Adaptive House. But iDorm learning system predefined fuzzy partition of each input space before learning. A properly divided fuzzy input space can reduce input complexity, but improperly and roughly divided fuzzy input space may hinder the knowledge acquiring process. Moreover, we have no feasible reason to divide input space into maximally specific fuzzy variable to explain human's corresponding action before learning.

For these reasons, FILS (Fuzzy Incremental Learning System)[16] has been proposed and applied for the virtual steward robot in the sense of constructing fuzzy partitions while extracting rules from training data. Figure 6 shows the learning procedure and illustrative example of FILS.

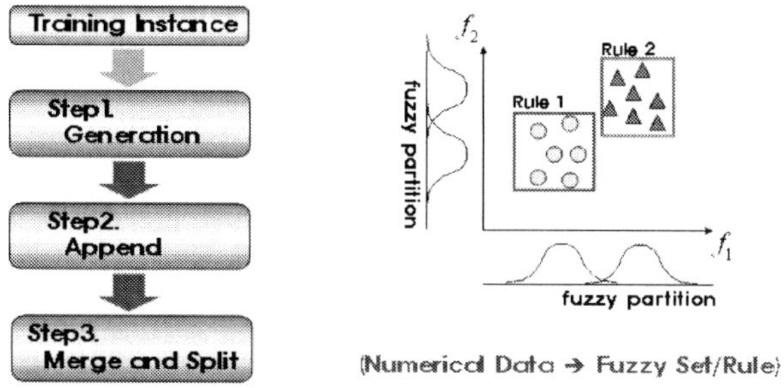

Figure 6. Learning procedure of FILS

Here, the learning procedure has been designed to minimize data-order dependency with statistical calculation. For given m attributes (sensory information) and n control outputs, m by n MIMO system should be represented as the collection of n MISO systems with m-input attributes at the initial stage. FILS transforms incrementally drawn training data into the corresponding fuzzy terms and association rules. After a certain time period, meaningful features are extracted by estimating PDF (probability density function) for each class and calculating the separabilty index of each PDF. Figure 7 shows feature selection diagram of the learning system.

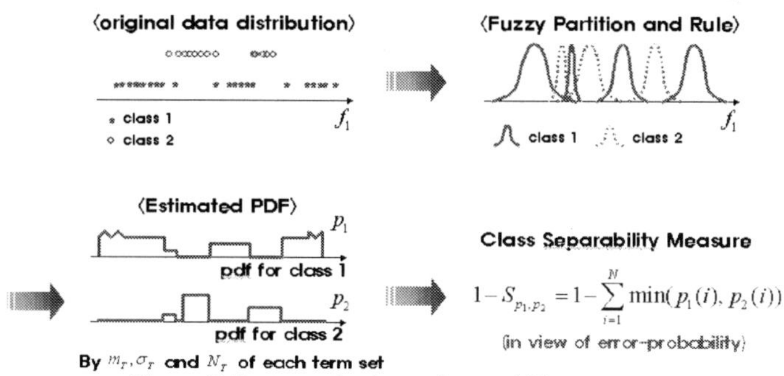

Figure 7. Feature selection and separability measure

Combining the above explained procedures, the overall learning structure is shown in the figure 8.

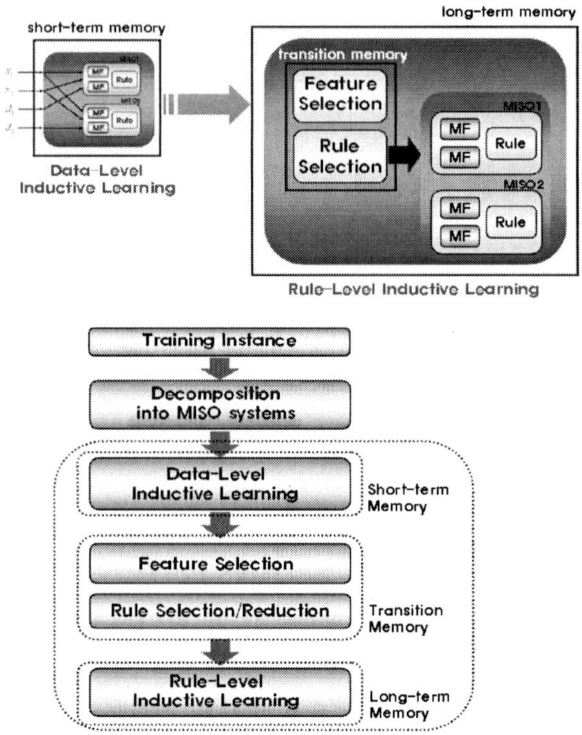

(a) Learning Structure (b) Learning Procedure

Figure 8. Overall learning structure and procedure

3. Realization of Hardware Type Steward Robot

The conceptual appearance design is as shown in the Figure 9. For this appearance design, Sasang Constitution Medical theory [17] has been utilized. Based on this theory, previous service robots are categorized into 4 predefined types (T'ae-yang-in, T'ae-eum-in, So-yang-in and So-eum-in), and then finally So-eum-in type has been selected for steward robot as an appearance type for human-friendly identity.

Figure 10 shows internal structure of the steward robot. Systems specification is as follows:

- 2 DOF for head motion
- 2 ×(6 DOF robot arm+1 DOF gripper)
- 2 wheel-driven mobile platform + 1 omni castor
- Ultrasonic sensor for navigation
- Recharging system
- 600mm×600mm×1100mm
- 2 CPU + 1 microprocessor
- wireless LAN/CAN(external/internal communication)

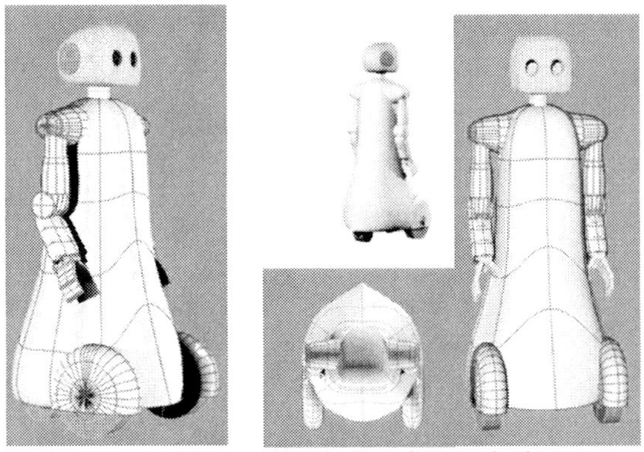

Figure 9. Conceptual design of steward robot

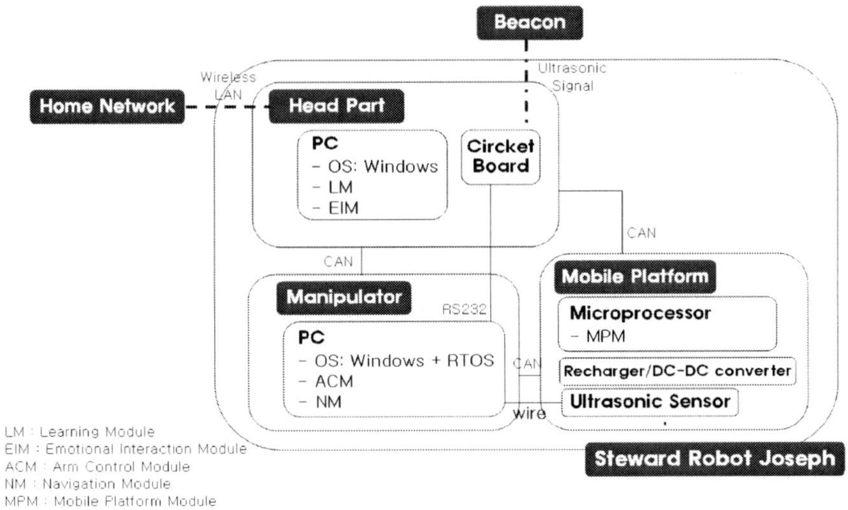

Figure 10. System structure

Functions of virtual Joseph are inherited into the head component. Emotional facial expressions are displayed using eyes, and management and task scheduling is done by the learning module. The control strategy of the two-armed manipulator is basically made in consideration of safety issue. Also, motion capture techniques are utilized to achieve smooth and natural motion trajectory of the robot arm. Localization of the mobile platform is accomplished using 3 beacons on the ceiling of the ISH for global path generation. Ultrasonic sensor is also used for collision avoidance. Regarding power supply, a mini DC-DC converter has been attached to each subsystem, and a recharging system with equalizer has been developed for efficient recharging of the battery.

4. Concluding Remarks

In this paper, we proposed a concept of a steward robot by which all services in a smart home can be provided appropriately and the subsystems can be controlled for each service. Also, learning and emotional interaction capabilities do an important role for steward robot to perform human-friendly interaction in the view of extended concept of service robot. The proposed steward robot will be helpful for older persons and people with disabilities by reducing the user cognitive load.

References

[1] Z. Zenn Bien, Kwang-Hyun Park, and Jin-Woo Jung, Intelligent Sweet Home - Welfare-Oriented Robotic House for Assisting the Handicapped and the Elderly, Proc. of ICRA 2004, New Orleans, LA, USA, April 2004

[2] Kim, Y., Park, K.–H., Seo, K.–H., Kim, C.H., Lee, W.–J., Song, W.–G., Do, J.–H., Lee, J.–J., Kim, B.K., Kim, J.–O., Lim, J.–T. and Bien, Z. "A report on questionnaire for developing Intelligent Sweet Home for the disabled and the elderly in Korean living conditions", Proceedings of the 8th International Conference on Rehabilitation Robotics, Daejeon, Korea, pp. 171-174.

[3] Meredith Faith, Julian F. Thayer, "A dynamical systems interpretation of a dimensional model of emotion", Scandinavian Journal of Psychology, Vol. 42, No. 121-133, 2001

[4] James A. Russell, "A Circumplex Model of Affect", Journal of Personality and Social Psychology, Vol. 39, No. 6, 1161-1178, 1980

[5 Kent E. Hutchison, et all, "A comparison of two models of emotion: Can measurement of emotion based on one model be used to make inferences about the other?", 1996

[6] Andrew Ortony, Gerald L. Clore, Allan Collins, "The Cognitive Structure of Emotions", Cambridge University Press, 1988

[7] D.A. Norman, A. Ortony, D.M. Russell, "Affect and machine design: Lessons for the development of autonomous machines", IBM Systems Journal 2003, Vol. 42, No. 1, pp. 38~44, 2003

[8] Christoph Bartneck, "Integrating the OCC Model of Emotions in Embodied Characters", 1998

[9] Cynthia Breazeal, "Function Meets Style : Insights from emotion theory applied to HRI", IEEE trans. SMC, Vol. 34, No. 2, 2004

[10] Hiroyasu Miwa, Tetsuya Okuchi, et all, "A New Mental Model of Humanoid Robots for Human Friendly Communication", Proc. Of the 2003 IEEE International Conference on R&A, Sep 14-19, 2003

[11] Bates, Joseph, "The role of emotion in believable agents", Association for Computing Machinery, Vol. 37, No. 7, pp. 122-126, 1994

[12] Mozer. M. C., "The neural network house: An environment that adapts to its inhabitants", Proc.of the American Association for Artificial Intelligence Spring Symposium on Intelligent Environments, Menlo, Park, pp. 110-114, 1998

[13] H. Hagras et. al, "Incremental Synchronous Learning for Embedded Agents Operating in Ubiquitous Computing Environments", Soft Computing Agents, IOS Press, pp. 25-55, 2002

[14] H. Duman, V. Callaghan, H. Hagras, M. Colley, G. Clarke, Z. Bien, H. Lee, Y. Kim "A Multi-Agent Pervasive Computing Architecture For Geographically Dispersed Care Environments" Proceedings of the 10th International Fuzzy Systems Association World Congress (IFSA 2003), Turkey 2003.

[15] U. Fayyad, G. Piatetsky-Shapiro, and P. Smyth, "From Data Mining to Knowledge Discovery: An Overview", in Advances in Knowledge Discovery and Data Mining, MIT Press, Cambridge, Mass., 1996, pp. 1-36.

[16] H. E. Lee, Y.M.Kim, J.W.Jung and Z. Zenn Bien, "Living behavior pattern learning system for human-friendly assistive home environment", International Conference on Smart Homes and Health Telematic 2005, Canada, pp.215-220

[17] The Association of Korean Oriental Medicine official site, http://www.akom.org/eng/theory/t1_2.htm

Promoting Independence for Older Persons with Disabilities
W.C. Mann and A. Helal (Eds.)
IOS Press, 2006

Development of Autonomous Robotic Wheelchair System

Chong Hui KIM [a,1], Seong Jin KIM [a], Hyun-Sang KIM [a], and Byung Kook KIM [a]
[a] *Dept. of EECS, Korea Advanced Institute of Science and Technology, Yuseong-gu, Daejeon, South Korea*

Abstract. Many people with mobility impairments have difficulty using ordinary wheelchairs for a variety of reasons. Powered wheelchairs can alleviate many inconveniences, but require battery charging and transferring between bed and wheelchair may be difficult. We developed a robotic wheelchair to resolve these problems. The robotic wheelchair can operate in three modes: manual, semi-autonomous, and autonomous. In autonomous mode, it can perform autonomous docking to both the battery charging station and the mechatronic transfer robot system.

Introduction

Powered wheelchairs are a widely used locomotive system for people with severe motor disabilities. Robotic wheelchairs have been the subject of intensive research activities. Representative research includes NavChair [3] and Smart Wheelchair Component System [4] in the USA, VAHM [5], SIAMO [6], MAid [7], and Rolland [8] in European Community, and KARES II [9] in South Korea. Few systems are commercially available [10]. Our preliminary survey with potential users [11] found that, most hesitate to employ a powered wheelchair because of tasks beyond their ability such as difficulty with transfers between wheelchair and bed, and cumbersome battery charging.

This paper presents our robotic wheelchair system developed by retrofitting a commercial powered wheelchair. It provides autonomous docking to both Mechatronic Transfer Robot (MTR) and Battery Charging Station (BCS). In Section 1 of this paper, we describe our hardware design including sensor system. Section 2 presents our software design for real-time capability under RTAI. Section 3 describes the algorithm for mobility and transfer aid and Section 4 shows the experimental results. Finally we conclude in Sections 5.

1. System Description

1.1. Hardware Design

The developed robotic wheelchair is based on a commercial powered wheelchair as shown in Figure 1. It is equipped with a PC mounted on the back of the wheelchair and operated on the RTAI, one of Linux real-time extension to provide real-time capability. It is also equipped with several sensors such as Laser Range Finder (LRF), wheel encoders, and instrumented bumper which are used for localization, obstacle detection, and collision detection for autonomy and safety.

Since many people with severe disabilities have difficulty controlling a powered wheelchair with a universal joystick, a touch sensitive LCD is attached at the right armrest as a visual input/output interface.

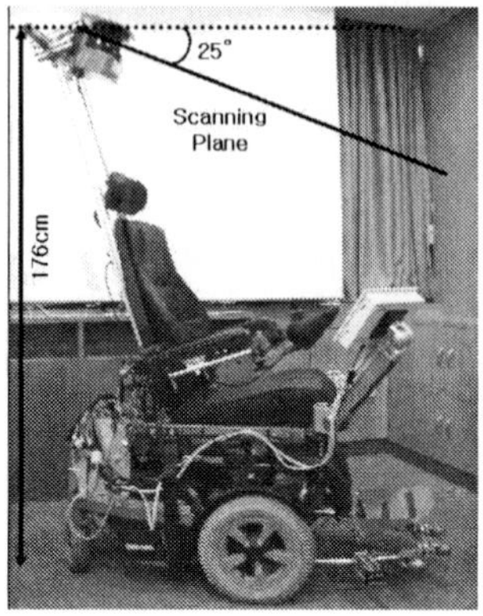

Figure 1. Robotic Wheelchair

The robotic wheelchair controller is divided into three components: PC, joystick module, and power module. The PC provides high-speed processing for control and data acquisition from sensors. The joystick and power modules are linked to the PC via RS232 serial ports, which permits the setting speed and steering angle every 10ms, as well as receiving the system's status.

1.2. Sensor System

The sensor system consists of two incremental encoders, LRF, and an instrumented bumper. The LRF is mounted on aluminum props at the height of 176cm and is inclined by 25 degrees as shown in Figure 1. Since it scans tilted plane from the height of LRF to the ground, it can detect obstacles below the height of the LRF without additional sensors, and 3-D environmental information can be obtained by accumulation of consecutive scanned 2-D plane images with movement of the wheelchair. Since a data packet for complete scan of the LRF is 733 bytes long, it is linked to the PC via a RS422 serial port for high speed data transmission at 500K bps. It scans the 180° coverage at 0.5° angular resolution in every complete scan time of 26ms.

Odometric measurements are obtained by two incremental encoders. These measurements are used to calculate the relative position and orientation of the wheelchair every 10ms.

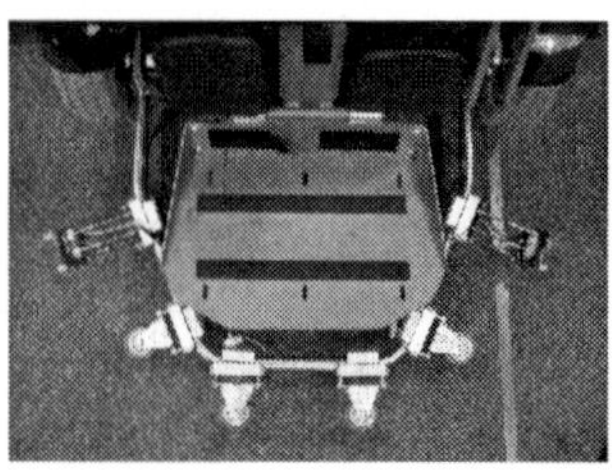

Figure 2. Instrumented Bumper

There is also an instrumented bumper for safe docking which consists of six sensing parts as shown in Figure 2. Each part is equipped with a micro-switch and a roller. It detects collisions with other objects, and also allows the robotic wheelchair to be docked quickly through gliding motion by rollers and using collision information by micro-switches.

2. Software Design for Robotic Wheelchair

2.1. Operation Modes

A robotic wheelchair can provide mobility and precise control which may be impossible or difficult for many powered wheelchair users. However, it does not exceed the perceptive and intellectual capability of humans. Our software has three operation modes: manual, semi-autonomous, and autonomous modes. In manual mode, a robotic wheelchair yields to the user's command via joystick or touch panel, except that it watches safety through environment perception. In semi-autonomous mode, the wheelchair is jointly controlled by the user and the computer to share environment perception and intelligence. If the user issues a command, wheelchair controller interprets the user's intention and evaluates risk using sensor information. If there are no risks, the intention is reflected in controlling a wheelchair. Otherwise, the wheelchair controller overrides the user's command to ensure safety. In autonomous mode, a robotic wheelchair carries out given missions using sensor information and its controller. In this mode, the robotic wheelchair can perform autonomous docking to both BCS and MTR. We designed the autonomous mode so that it automatically changes to semi-autonomous mode whenever there is any command from the user.

In order to provide mobility assistance, we defined eight operation states as shown in Figure 3. Each operation state is very complex since it consists of various tasks such as localization, navigation, object detection, path planning, and motor control. Timely correctness of each task is important for ensuring the safety of the user.

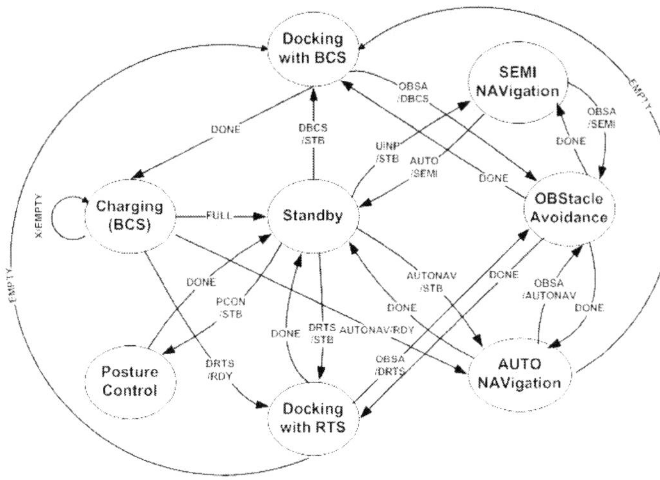

Figure 3. State Diagram of Operation

2.2. Real-Time Software Architecture

Our control architecture has a hierarchical structure as shown in Figure 4. The controller has three layers. The bottom layer performs low-level motor control and position feedback from encoders at every T_{MOTOR} period. The middle control layer solves tasks related to environment sensing, localization, object detection, obstacle avoidance, localization, and trajectory following during T_{LRF} periods. The tasks that this layer solves require much higher computational resources than those of the bottom layer. The top layer addresses tasks such as selection of movement strategy and trajectory planning that are executed sporadically.

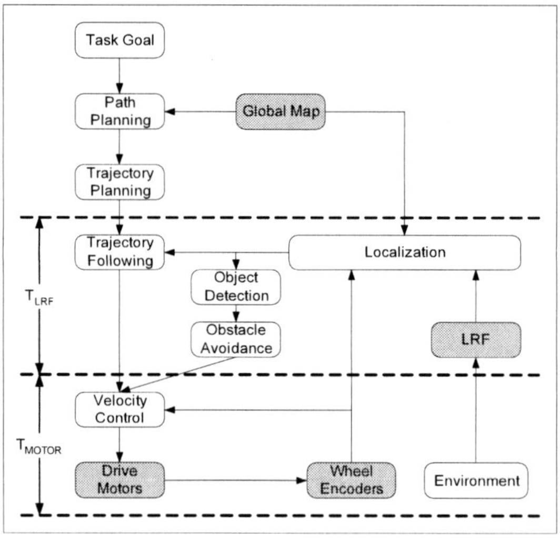

Figure 4. Hierarchical Control Architecture

Wheelchair safety in automatic mode depends on a timely response for each task. If the sensor information is delayed, obstacles will be detected too late and a collision may occur. The problem can be solved by using real-time computation in the bottom and middle layers where the information from the sensors and actuators is processed. In our design, we used Linux with real-time extension RTAI (Real-Time Application Interface), since it is free software with open source code and offers a comprehensive development environment including debugger and graphical user interface.

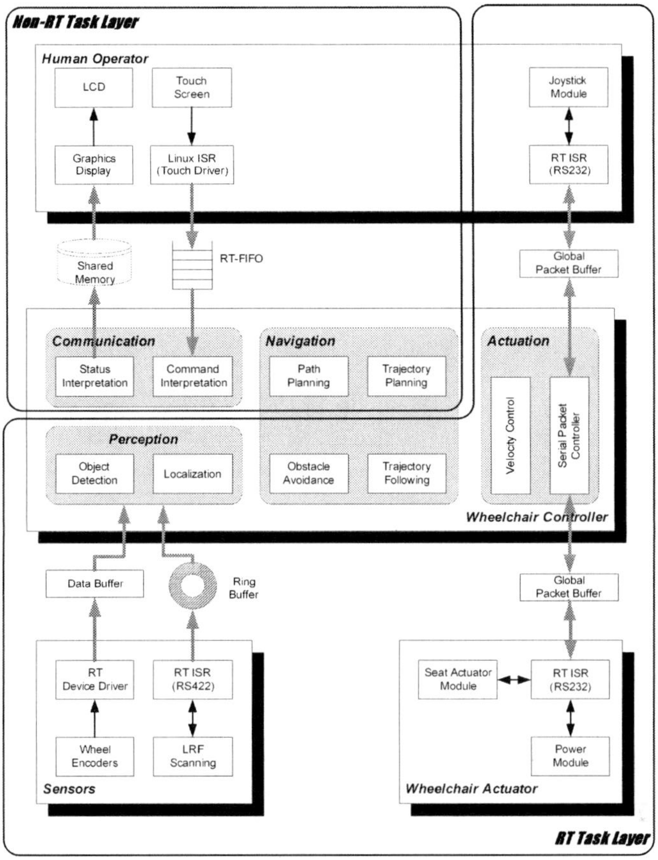

Figure 5. Software Architecture of Developed Robotic Wheelchair

The software architecture of our system has two layers as shown in Figure 5. The RT task layer deals with tasks such as motor control and perception which require strict in-time real-time computation. The Non-RT task layer is responsible for the graphical user interface and handles navigation tasks such as path planning, and also processes user's commands, of which their execution times are not constrained. Tasks between two layers communicate by means of shared memory and RT-FIFO.

3. Mobility and Transfer Aid

Most people who use a powered wheelchair have difficulty transferring between bed and wheelchair, and battery charging. Autonomous transferring and battery charging are most important functionalities of a wheelchair for increasing independence. Our robotic wheelchair can provide autonomous transfer aid and autonomous battery charging as well as mobility. For autonomous battery charging and transfer assistance, the robotic wheelchair is trying to dock with BCS (Figure 6) and MTR (Figure 7).

The basic idea is based on the localization and the pose estimation using object detection from 2-D scan data of LRF [12, 13]. The docking process has three phases:

(1) Approaching phase - moving to the predefined docking ready position, (2) Pose estimation phase - estimating the pose of target system (MTR or BCS), (3) Docking phase - docking with target system performing position control for complete docking.

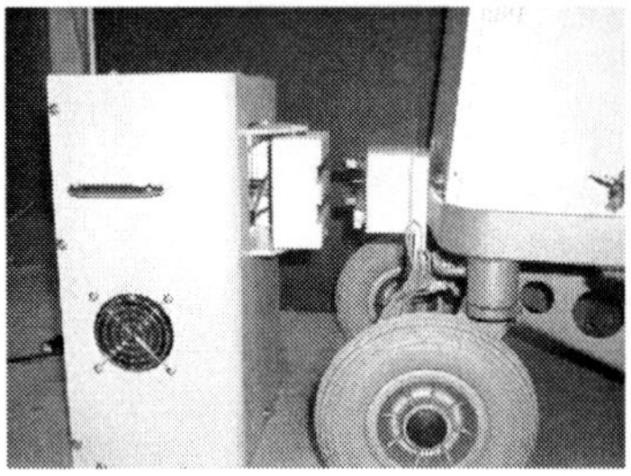

Figure 6. Battery Charging Station

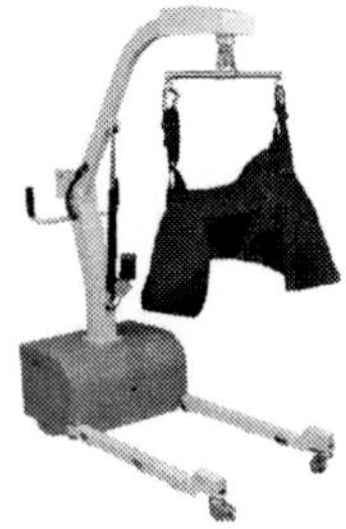

Figure 7. Mechatronic Transfer Robot

In the following subsections, we explain our localization algorithm and docking strategy with MTR.

3.1. Localization

Our localization algorithm is based on line feature and map matching. Since the LRF provides clear line features for an indoor environment, lines provide strong and accurate information, but with far fewer points. Therefore, line based algorithms are more appropriate for the real-time processing compared to algorithms that are point based. Localization is performed in four steps.

- **Step 1:** Extract line segments from the scan data using the recursive line splitting method [14].
- **Step 2:** Fit the splitted lines into lines with least square error, and project start and end points of segments on the corresponding line.
- **Step 3:** Estimate the position of wheelchair in world coordinates by identifying matched pairs.
- **Step 4:** Find the matching pairs of line segments between the given map and sensed data.

From the matching result, the robotic wheelchair localizes its position by minimizing the following proposed cost function. Let G_i and M_k be a matching pair as shown in Figure 8, where G_i is an ith segmented scan data with N_i scan points and M_k is global map line segments defined by polar coordinates with start and end points. Let d_{ij} be the perpendicular distance from a data point of G_i to the map line segment M_k, l_i be the length of the data line segment L_i, and σ_i^2 be the variance of the distances between data points G_i and the data line segment L_i.

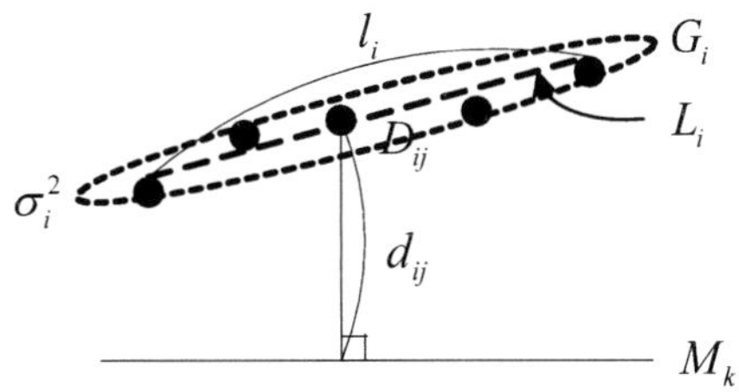

Figure 8. Parameters for Line Segment Matching

When ϕ and $P=[p_x\ p_y]^T$ are defined as rotation angle and translation vector respectively, d_{ij} is a function of ϕ and P. The proposed cost function using $d_{ij}(\phi, P)$ is

$$E(\phi,P)=\sum_{i=1}^{N_s}\frac{l_i}{\sigma_i^2}\sum_{j=1}^{N_i}d_{ij}^2(\phi,P) \tag{1}$$

where l_i/σ_i^2 is additional weight of G_i which means that a segment with longer length and less variance is more reliable.

The term $d_{ij}^2(\phi,P)$ can be expanded as

$$d_{ij}^2(\phi,P)=\left[m_i\left(\Delta_{ij}\Phi+P\right)-\rho_i^M\right]^2 \tag{2}$$

where

$$m_i=\begin{bmatrix}\cos\theta_i^M & \sin\theta_i^M\end{bmatrix},\ \Delta_{ij}=\begin{bmatrix}x_{ij} & -y_{ij}\\ y_{ij} & x_{ij}\end{bmatrix},\text{ and }\Phi=\begin{bmatrix}\cos\phi\\ \sin\phi\end{bmatrix}$$

Then the equation (1) has the extended form by equation (2) as follows:

$$E(\Phi,P)=\Phi^T\mathbf{A}\Phi+2\mathbf{P}^T\mathbf{B}\Phi+\mathbf{P}^T\mathbf{C}\mathbf{P}-2\mathbf{U}^T\Phi-2\mathbf{V}^T\mathbf{P}+k \tag{3}$$

All local minima of equation (3) should satisfy the following set of equations:

$$\frac{E(\Phi,P)}{\partial\Phi}=\frac{E(\Phi,P)}{\partial P}=0 \tag{4}$$

From the equation (4), it is possible to express P as a function of Φ:

$$P=\mathbf{C}^{-1}\left(\mathbf{V}-\mathbf{B}\Phi\right) \tag{5}$$

If all matched map segments are almost parallel to each other, matrix **C** is nearly singular. Hence our localization algorithm is divided into two cases: (1) matrix **C** is nonsingular and (2) matrix **C** is singular.

(1) When matrix C is nonsingular - In this case, we can get a unique solution solving equation (3) as follows:

$$E(\Phi)=\Phi^T\mathbf{F}\Phi+2\mathbf{W}^T\Phi+k' \tag{6}$$

where

$$\mathbf{F} = \mathbf{A} - \mathbf{B}^T\mathbf{C}^{-T}\mathbf{B}, \ \mathbf{W} = \mathbf{B}^T\mathbf{C}^{-T}\mathbf{V} - \mathbf{U}, \text{ and } k' = k - \mathbf{V}^T\mathbf{C}^{-T}\mathbf{V}$$

Then E becomes a 2nd order polynomial of cos ø and sin ø with the constraint $\cos^2$ ø + $\sin^2$ ø = 1. According to Lagrange's theorem [15], it can be converted into a 4th order equation of cos ø or sin ø. By using several constraints [16], the answer is obtained.

(2) When matrix C is singular - This case usually happens in corridor navigation. Figure 9 describes an example with all matched map segments (M_2, M_3) parallel. In po sition computation, we can not obtain the unique solution since matrix **C** is singular. In this case, we can obtain the lateral position and orientation of wheelchair. By finding th e nearest point from the robotic position O by odometer, we consider the point P as the real robot position.

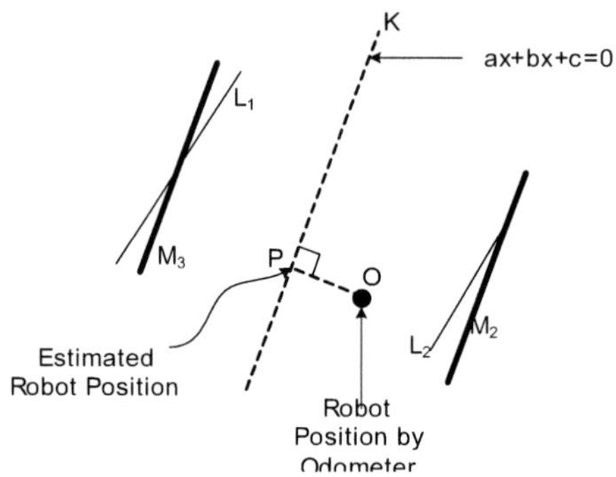

Figure 9. Localization when all matched map segments are parallel

From equation (4), we can get the following equation.

$$\mathbf{B}\Phi + \mathbf{C}P - \mathbf{V} = 0 \quad (7)$$

Since the matrix $\boldsymbol{C}$ is singular, P can not have a unique solution. To solve this problem, we change matrix $\boldsymbol{B}$ and $\boldsymbol{C}$ as follows:

$$\mathbf{C} = \begin{bmatrix} a & c \\ c & b \end{bmatrix} \text{ and } \mathbf{B} = \begin{bmatrix} d & e \\ \dfrac{cd}{a} & \dfrac{c}{a}e \end{bmatrix}$$

From equation (7), a line equation corresponding to line K is obtained:

$$dx + ey + ap_1 + cp_1 - v_1 = 0 \quad (8)$$

Next, use of the following Lagrange equation has the constraint $\Phi^T\Phi = 1$, we obtain the rotation vector Φ.

$$H = E(\Phi, P) + \lambda(\Phi^T\Phi - 1) \quad (9)$$

3.2. Pose Estimation for Docking Process

Since the docking position and the pose of MTR vary near the predefined docking ready position, the exact position and the pose of MTR are required for safe docking. To obtain the required docking information, a key idea is to detect the legs of MTR using LRF and estimate the pose of MTR using the structural dimension feature of MTR. Pose estimation of MTR has four steps:

- Step 1: Detect object from LRF scan data.
- Step 2: Find leg candidates from objects satisfying structural feature of MTR.
- Step 3: Move forward to get accumulated leg information.
- Step 4: Estimate the pose from accumulated leg information using least square fit.

At Step 1, we perform the object detection from LRF scan data. For the segmentation of scan data, we used Castro's method [17]. At Step 2, we choose objects from the segment group and save the center of the segment satisfying four conditions as the leg of MTR:

i) The number of points of a segment is greater than three points, which is the necessary condition to be a candidate of the object.
ii) The number of points of the segment is less than six points which equals to t he thickness of the leg (about 50mm).
iii) The height of a segment to the ground is in the range between 110mm and 1 50mm, since the height of the leg is 130mm from the ground.
iv) Relative distance of the segment from the center along the lateral direction i s less than 1000mm considering the structural feature of MTR.

To acquire the accumulated leg information, at Step 3, the robotic wheelchair moves forward incrementally with open-loop control until 100 scan data are gathered. It takes about 2.6s to get the 100 scan data since every complete scan time of LRF is about 26ms. Finally, we estimate the pose of MTR from accumulated leg information using the least square fit.

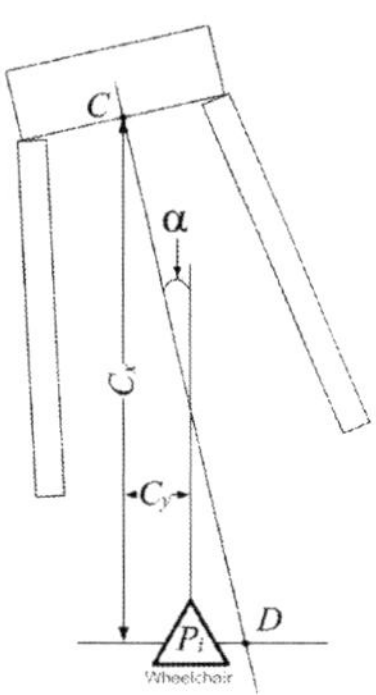

Figure 10. Pose Estimation Model

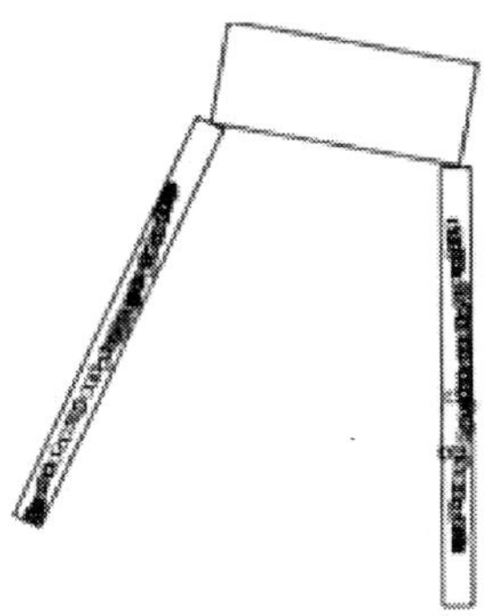

Figure 11. Accumulated Leg Data

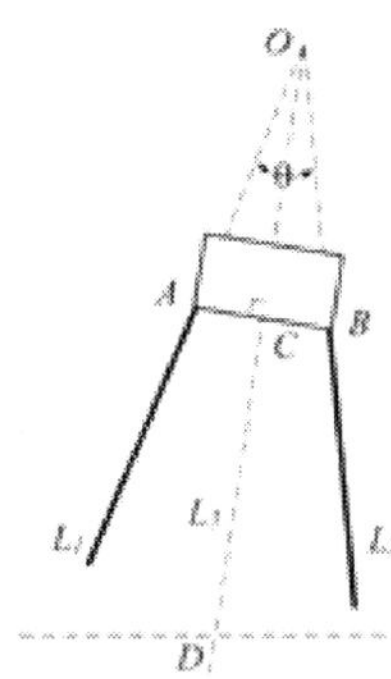

Figure 12. Geometry Model

From the accumulated leg information as shown in Figure 11, we can estimate the pose (C_x, C_y, α) of MTR with respect to the robotic wheelchair (see Figure 10). Using least square fit, we can get the estimate line segment L_1 and L_2 of each leg as shown in Figure 12. Each line segment has the following forms:

$$y_1 = a_1 x_1 + b_1 \text{ and } y_2 = a_2 x_2 + b_2 \tag{10}$$

Then we can get the angle θ between L_1 and L_2, and inclined angle a_3 of L_3 to find the center of base of MTR $\left(\overline{AB}\right)$.

$$\theta = tan^{-1}\left(\frac{a_2 - a_1}{1 + a_1 a_2}\right) \text{ and } a_3 = \frac{tan(\theta/2) + a_1}{1 - a_1 tan(\theta/2)} \tag{11}$$

Hence the estimated position of MTR is obtained as follows:

$$C_x = \frac{\left(\overline{OD} - \overline{OC}\right)x_0 + \overline{OC}x_d}{\overline{OD}}, \quad C_y = \frac{\left(\overline{OD} - \overline{OC}\right)y_0}{\overline{OD}} \text{ and}$$

$$\alpha = atan2\left(1, \frac{1}{a_3}\right) - \frac{\pi}{2} \tag{12}$$

where C=(C_x, C_y) is the center of body of MTR, C=(x_d, 0) is the center of robotic wheelchair, and O=(x_0, y_0) is the intersection of lines L_1 and L_2.

4. Experiments

We tested the robotic wheelchair at *Intelligent Sweet Home* in KAIST. In order to verify the localization algorithm, we performed the following experiment: the robotic wheelchair was navigated to an arbitrary path and returned to the start point. We compared two results using both LRF and odometer, and using odometer only. When we use both LRF and odometer, as shown in Figure 13, the end point was nearly the same as the start point. When we use odometer only, however, the end point is not the same as the start point as shown in Figure 14. Hence localization failed and accumulated error is increased with traveling distance.

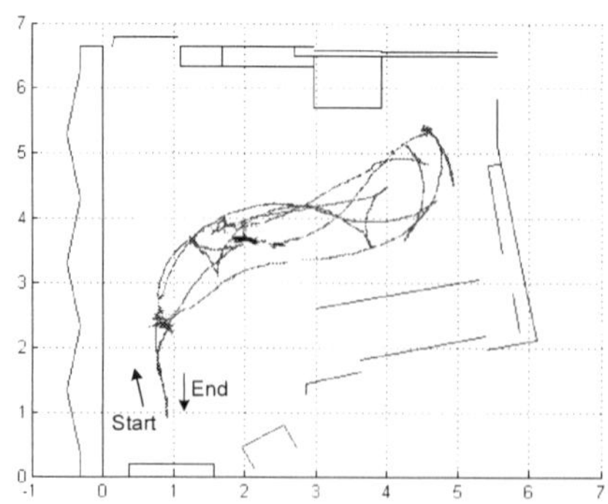

Figure 13 Localization using LRF and Odometer

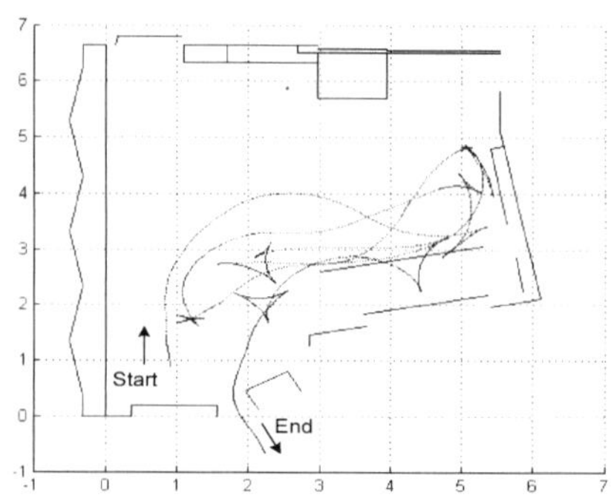

Figure 14 Localization using odometer only

We also experimented with the docking mechanism for transfers between wheelchair and bed. Figure 15 shows the pose estimation result during transfer assistance (**x** denotes the estimated position and **o** denotes the real position of MTR). The accuracy of the estimated position of MTR shows ± 100mm for position and ± 4° for orientation.

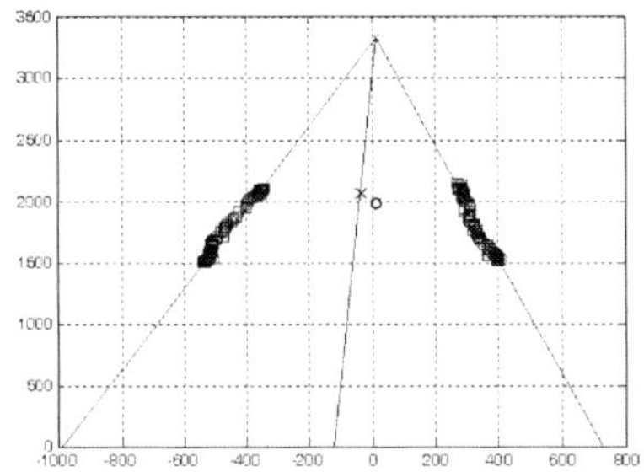

Figure 15. Localization using LRF and Odometer

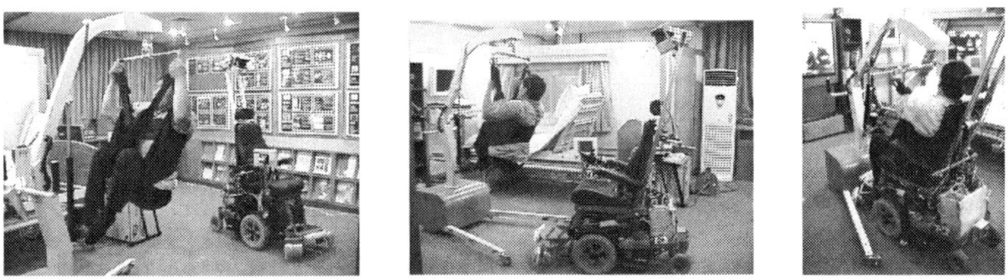

(a) Approaching Phase (b) Pose Estimation Phase (c) Docking Phase

Figure 16. Docking Process for Transferring between wheelchair and bed

During the docking, all tasks of the robotic wheelchair were done in real-time without missing deadline as shown in Table 1.

Table 1. Execution Time of Each Task

Module	Task	Worse Execution Time	Deadline
Motor	Motor Control	0.46ms	2.0ms
	RS422 Data Tx.	16.5ms	
	Feature Extraction	0.49ms	
Navigation	Map Matching	0.35ms	26.0ms
	Object Detection	0.35ms	
	Location Update	0.08ms	
Docking	Pose Estimation	0.46ms	10.0ms
Bumper	Bumper Handling	0.05ms	

5. Conclusion

We developed a robotic wheelchair for people with severe motor impairment which can provide mobility and transfer assistance with manual, semi-autonomous, and autonomous operation modes. For real-time processing, we adopted Linux with RTAI and control software under RTAI. To provide mobility assistance, we developed a localization algorithm using LRF and validated the performance with the result of using odometer only. We also carried out experiments with potential user with motor disabilities in Intelligent Sweet Home at KAIST so that our developed robotic wheelchair could navigate and dock with MTR, and assist with transfers between wheelchair and bed.

Acknowledgement

This work is fully supported by KOSEF through HWRS-ERC at KAIST. The authors are grateful to Prof. Jin-Oh Kim who developed the mechatronic transfer robot system. We also thank Kwang-Suk Seo for his participation in testing.

References

[1] S. Fioretti, T. Leo, and S. Longhi, "A Navigation System for Increasing Autonomy and the Security of Powered Wheelchairs," *IEEE Transactions on Rehabilitation Engineering*, vol. 8, no. 4, 2000, pp. 490-498

[2] Kwang-Hyun Park and Z. Zenn. Bien, "Intelligent Sweet Home for Assisting the Elderly and the Handicapped," *1st International Conference on Smart Homes and Health Telematics*, France, 2004, pp. 151-158

[3] Simpson P. Levine, David A. Bell, Lincoln A. Jaros, Richard C. Simpson, Yoram Koren, and Johan Borenstein, "The NavChair Assistive Wheelchair Navigation System," *IEEE Transactions on Rehabilitation Engineering*, vol. 7, no. 4, 1999, pp. 443-451

[4] Richard Simpson, Edmund LoPresti, Illah Nourbakhsh, and David Miller, "The Smart Wheelchair Component System," *Journal of Rehabilitation Research and Development*, vol. 41, no. 38, 2004, pp. 429-442

[5] G. Bourhis, O. Horn, O. Havert, and A. Pruski, "An Autonomous Vehicle for People with Motor Disabilities," *IEEE Robotics and Automation Magazine*, vol. 8, no. 1, 2001, pp. 57-65

[6] Manuel Mazo et al., "An Integral System for Assisted Mobility," *IEEE Robotics and Automation Magazine*, vol. 8, no. 1, 2001, pp. 46-56

[7] Erwin Prassler, Jens Scholz, and Paolo Fiorini, "A Robotics Wheelchair for Crowded Public Environments," *IEEE Robotics and Automation Magazine*, vol. 8, no. 1, 2001, pp. 38-45

[8] Axel Lankenau and Thomas Röfer, "A Versatile and Safe Mobility Assistance," *IEEE Robotics and Automation Magazine*, vol. 8, no. 1, 2001, pp. 29-37

[9] Zenn. Bien, Dae-Jin Kim, Myung-Jin Chung, Dong-Soo Kwon, Pyung-Hun Chang, "Development of a Wheelchair-Based Rehabilitation Robotic System (KARES II) with Various Human-Robot Interaction Interfaces for the Disabled," *IEEE/ASME International Conference on Advanced Intelligent Mechatronics*, vol. 2, 2003, pp. 902-907

[10] Paul D. Nisbelt, "Who's intelligent? Wheelchair, driver or both?," *IEEE International Conference on Control Applications*, 2002, pp. 760-765.

[11] Chong Hui Kim, Jik Han Jung, and Byung Kook Kim, "Design of Intelligent Wheelchair for the Motor Disabled," *8th International Conference on Rehabilitation* Robotics, Daejeon, South Korea, 2003, pp. 92-95

[12] Chong Hui Kim, Seong Jun Kim, Sang Woo Choi, and Byung Kook Kim, "Development of a Real-Time Control System for Powered Wheelchair using Laser Range Finder," *The 5th International Workshop on Human-friendly Welfare Robotic Systems*, April 2004, pp. 10-15

[13] Chong Hui Kim, Seong Jin Kim, and Byung Kook Kim, "Pose Estimation and Docking of Robotic Wheelchair to Robotic Transfer System for Autonomous Transfer Aid of Motor-Disabled," *8th European Conference for the Advancement of Assistive Technology in Europe (AAATE2005)*, September 2005, pp. 317-321

[14] L. Zhang and B. K. Ghosh, "Line Segment Based Map Building and Localization using 2D Laser Range Finder," *IEEE International Conference on Robotic and Automation*, vol. 3, 20000, pp. 2538-2543

[15] K. P. Chong and H. Zak, *An Introduction to Optimization*, 2nd Edition, John Wiley & Sons, 2001

[16] Hee Jin Sohn and Byung Kook Kim, "A Robust Localization Algorithm for Mobile Robots with Laser Range Finders," IEEE International Conference on Robotics and Automation, 2005, pp. 102-107

[17] D. Castro, U. Nunes, and A. Runao, "Reactive Local Navigation," IEEE 28th Annual Conference on Industrial Electronics Society, 2002, pp. 2427-2432.

Chapter 2

Telehealth

Promoting Independence for Older Persons with Disabilities
W.C. Mann and A. Helal (Eds.)
IOS Press, 2006

Attention Care and Monitoring of Behavior

Charles WILLEMS[a,1], Frank VLASKAMP[a], and Suzanne DE VLIEGER[a]
[a]*Institute for Rehabilitation Research iRv, Hoensbroek The Netherlands*

Abstract. In an implementation project in The Netherlands a small investigation was made of the most urgent needs of older home care clients. Two potential user groups for the development of specific care-arrangements were indicated: "older persons becoming lonely and inactive", and "partners/caregivers of patients with dementia." The care-arrangement "Attention Care" is aimed at supporting lonely persons and the care-arrangement "Monitoring of Behavior" is aimed at providing surveillance at a distance to support the care giving relative of a person with dementia. Both care arrangements use video telephony to communicate with professional caregivers. In February 2005, field trials started, which will continue until the end of November 2005. Evaluation of data gathered during this trial is discussed.

Keywords. Home care, care at a distance, information and communication technologies, dementia, loneliness

Introduction

In the Netherlands care for older persons at home is delivered by home care organizations and as a service to the community from homes for the elderly and nursing homes. The use of specific information and communication technologies (ICT) for the contact between clients at home and the care centre is limited to emergency response systems.

Some organizations providing care at home are developing 24 hour-a-day services. In the project ICT-Unplannable Care, several care organizations joined forces to provide home care services at night and weekends. This service is accessed via telephone [1]. The contact between the caller and the caregiver is limited to exchanging information about the emergency and the help that is needed.

Some care organizations are aware that ICT may have an important role in the care process itself [2,3,4]. Pilots have been initiated to gather knowledge on the opportunities and required conditions to implement ICT in the delivery of care. In this paper the development and pilot implementation of the newly defined care programs "Attention Care" and "Monitoring behavior" are discussed.

1. Selection of care arrangements

The core business of organizations providing care at home lies in nursing care, personal care, housekeeping services, monitoring of patients, special care in case of social or psychological problems, information provision and provision of assistive technology. Many of these care services require face-to-face contact between caregiver and client and presence of a caregiver at home. Some services seem to be suited for care at a distance, such as care for persons with psychological problems and patient monitoring. Several interviews with health care professionals were held and a workshop with home care workers was organized to identify potential care arrangements in which ICT could be used [5]. As a result, two care arrangements were selected for further development: "Attention Care" and "Monitoring of Behavior." Both care arrangements address the problems of a large potential user group, and video contact may be an efficient way to be "present" in the home of a client when support and assistance is needed. In cooperation with two organizations a pilot study was initiated. In this investigation the conditions to deliver the respective care arrangements were identified and organized. Technology was selected based on an inquiry of technology already available in the market. Criteria to select clients were determined.

1.1. Attention Care

The care arrangement "Attention Care" is available for older persons with feelings of loneliness, loss of control, and lack of initiative. The purpose of the care arrangement is to stimulate the client to be active again and to regain control of his/her own life. A professional contact person seeks video-telephone contact with the client on pre-arranged moments (for instance: twice a week). The client can also initiate a call to talk with the contact person. In the clients' house an IP broadband video telephone is installed [6].

The video telephone can be operated hands free. Optionally, the video telephone can be connected to a set of wireless speakers and an extra microphone. The size of the color video screen on the telephone is 10 by 7,5 cm, the use of the TV as a large display is an option. The caregiver at the care centre has the same video telephone configuration. Additionally, the caregiver has a PC database for registration and planning of calls.

1.2. Monitoring of Behaviour

The care arrangement "Monitoring of Behavior" is available for the partner or informal caregivers of a patient with (early) dementia who is still living at home. The purpose of this care arrangement is to support the partner or informal caregiver. If the partner or informal caregiver wants to leave the house, he or she calls the care centre, and informs the care centre that surveillance is wanted. Monitoring is not possible all the time, and has to be arranged before with the client (for instance: a monitoring session of an hour on 1-3 afternoons per week).

The caregiver at the care centre has a PC with a color monitor that displays images from up to 4 surveillance cameras in the patient's house. It is also possible to talk and listen to the patient. Another PC handles the information from sensors. The caregiver at the care centre is alerted when a potentially dangerous situation in the patient's house is detected, such as: smoke, patient is wandering, loud noise, etc. The patient or informal caregiver can also take the initiative to alert the care centre. Pressing the (portable) alarm button of a care telephone sends a distress call to the care center.

The care arrangement includes a quick response time: within 20 minutes after detecting a dangerous situation or receiving a distress call a professional care worker is present at the home of the patient. The caregiver at the care centre can also call the ambulance, doctor, or the fire brigade when needed. To facilitate access, the front door is equipped with an electronic lock, that can be remotely opened by a signal from the care centre.

The partner or informal caregiver of the dementia patient can consult an expert (geriatric nurse) to talk about problems related to dementia and care for a dementia patient. Consults take place via videoconferencing. The technology involved in setting up this care arrangement is put in a "toolbox," which contains 4 video cameras, 2 door sensors, 1 smoke sensor, 2 movement detectors, 1 bed rest sensor, 1 audio sensor. Based on an evaluation of the client's situation the technology required to support the care arrangement "Monitoring Behavior" is selected and installed.

2. Implementation and evaluation

In February 2005, the care organizations participating in the project started with the introduction of the care arrangements to their clients [7]. The number of clients participating in the pilot is 20 for "Attention Care" and 20 for "Monitoring of Behavior." An evaluation study :

- Defined the conditions under which care organizations can deliver the care arrangements "Attention Care" and "Monitoring of Behavior" as a routine health care product.
- Described how the care arrangements are used.
- Defined the user groups of "Attention Care" and "Monitoring of Behavior."
- Gave an indication of the cost of "Attention Care" and "Monitoring of Behavior."

3. Results

3.1. Attention Care

Both organizations were successful in selecting the clients for Attention Care. Within 3 months, both had selected at least 10 clients who agreed to participate. Major problems were encountered with the amount of technical support required in the house. Especially the realization of the IP broadband infrastructure caused a significant delay. In an interview before the start of the service clients were asked about their expectations of the service. All stated to have few social contacts. They expected that the video conversation would deal with a variety of subjects; the past, children, personal health, the health of their partner. Some indicated reservations: the subjects to be discussed would be influenced by the person at the other side of the videophone. After a period of use of 3 month on the average again an interview was done. (At the time this paper is written the evaluations of 6 clients are completed; services and data collection are still in progress). Out of the six clients interviewed in the second period two had a video conversation more than once a week. Four out of 6 clients stated that the video conversation has supported to reach the personal goals set in advance. Two clients indicated a negative result. When asked to rate personal well-being at a scale of 0-100 only small changes were noted: 2 clients indicated an increase of 10 points, 2 clients indicated no difference and 2 clients indicated a decrease of 10 points.

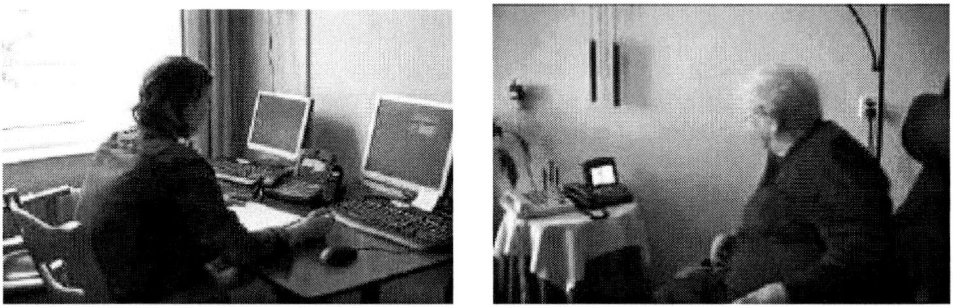

Figure 1. Infrastructure present at care center (left) and one client (right) in use to provide attention care.

During this evaluation period 11 clients actually had used Attention care. 24 different care providers are involved. In that period 142 contacts were recorded with an average length of 24 min. Subjects discussed were recorded in a database for later analysis. Subjects involved are daily activities and personal health (both 36%), social contacts (28%), specific task performance (23%), recreational activities (16%) and independence (8%) (more than one item per conversation could be scored).

Both clients and health care providers encountered problems in having this kind of conversation. The additional value of the video-image is at present difficult to determine. Care providers found it difficult to structure the conversation towards care related guidance. Clients expressed difficulties to value the conversations as care provision. In part this could be introduced by the fact that these video conversations are performed by appointment, in part also that they have a preset time interval of 30 minutes. In the second half of the pilot care providers will investigate the value of more frequent, but shorter video conversations (3-4 times a week for 10 min instead of once for 30 min).

3.2. Monitoring behavior (results)

The exact conditions under which Monitoring Behavior is delivered are determined in interaction with the client. Based on an assessment of the client system (housing plan, risk analysis of clients' behavior, potential interventions by the caregiver that can be done during monitoring sessions) the conditions of the care arrangement are specified. Also the technology is selected from the "toolbox" and installed in the house. Both the care provider and the partner of the clients were highly favored the use of video camera's to monitor the situation at a distance. The use of sensors (that would alert the care provider in case a unwanted situation would occur) was rejected. Since the cameras are only used during a monitoring session no privacy problems were encountered. During a typical monitoring session the partner of the client would leave the apartment for about 2 hrs. In that period care providers can only respond to the visual impressions unless the sensors are installed and used. Based this practical experience a renewed assessment of the client situation was organized. As a result thereof the use of sensors to support the monitoring process is stimulated. Also the monitoring of multiple situations has been introduced. In the beginning the monitoring process was performed by a selected group of 3 care workers. For practical reasons this group was expanded almost immediately after the start of the service delivery. For the monitoring of 7 clients in 50 sessions a total of 13 care workers were involved. During 50 monitoring sessions 3 incidents occurred that required an intervention by the care provider. Protocols how to handle in those situations were present and ranged from using voice communication to comfort the client and to alert a relative to visit the client. At the onset and during the pilot interviews were held with the partner of the client. After 3 month practice again interviews were held with 4 participants. All indicated in the beginning that they expected to become able to take up their own activities (Shopping, social contacts) during the monitoring period. Until that moment this was only possible in exceptional circumstances. During the second interview all indicated that the monitoring of their partner by care workers felt as a relief. They were able to perform their own activity knowing that the partner was under good surveillance. The incidents that happened were also noted in these interviews. These clients are positive about the service. The reaction of the patients with dementia could not be recorded directly since they could not be interviewed.

The care providers can only rely on the video image to monitor the situation at home since the sensors have not been introduced. During an intermediate review with the care providers the reasons for not suggesting these sensors as part of the care arrangement was discussed. This resulted in the proposal to re-assess the client situation to determine what sensors can be introduced to support the monitoring. At present the results of this re-assessment are not available.

4. Discussion

"Attention Care" and "Monitoring of Behavior" are new care arrangements, aimed for lonely elderly and the support of partners and caregivers of dementia patients. Loneliness in old age and dementia are huge problems for the clients involved and for society. The provision of support and surveillance at home for this large group is a time-consuming task which is too costly for health insurance. Home care volunteers are not always available. Care at a distance may be the solution [8].

In this pilot the care arrangements are formulated starting from the perspective an existing client – care provider relation. Until now, technology does not play a role in regular practice. Thus, both the client and the care provider needed to get used to the technology. Defining a care arrangement in practice may then become a difficult situation. Only in an environment in which this kind of "experimentation" is stimulated, real progress can be made. Within this project only technology already available on the market is used. However, video telephony via broadband IP connection is a relatively new technology. Thus a situation easily occurs that the conditions under which the technology actually become available have a great impact on the care arrangement that is actually implemented. In this pilot we have noted an unfortunate delay in the delivery of the IP broadband connections and a (in view of the clients and the care providers) a complicated functioning of the sensors. This resulted in a difference in the care arrangements that were intended to use and those actually used.

A second observation that can be made at this point is that it is difficult to convince care providers as well as clients to participate in an investigation like this. Both are reluctant to enter. These initial hesitations can be reduced if good results can be demonstrated based on pilot implementation. Consequently, implementation of new health care arrangements does require a good communication of initial results, both to clients and care providers [9].

It is not an easy task for a care organization to be innovative. When developing a new care arrangement, care organizations have to deal with the small margins in available personnel, tight budgets, strict health insurance rules and rigid structures in health care.

Innovative ideas often do not get the chance to prove their value. With this technology it becomes possible to maintain a low-cost video-connection with reasonable quality. The potential of sensor technology is great, in recent year's sensors and video cameras became cheap, easy-to-install and wireless. The technology is now readily available, and, potentially, it can help care organizations to develop innovative care arrangements. Implementing new care arrangements, however, is a challenge for the care organizations involved. It is the implementation of new technology, and - more important – it is a further step in health care renewal. Innovative care organizations like the ones participating in the project have to put a lot of energy in the development of new care arrangements.

Meanwhile, the use of mobile video telephones is growing at a rapid pace in the mainstream area. Telecom providers, such as Vodafone, are investing large amounts of money in the deployment of UMTS networks and in making this technology accessible and affordable for a large audience. The home care sector lags far behind in investments and use of new technology. And, more important, it lags behind in the development of useful applications. It will not take long before clients will expect that caregivers communicate in the same way with them as they do communicate with relatives and friends. Taking that into account, care organizations should not wait for that moment, but work on innovative concepts for providing care to persons who need it.

Acknowledgements

This implementation project is supported by a grant from the Province of Limburg in The Netherlands. The authors present this paper on behalf of the Steering Committee "ICT Unplannable Care." The project is carried out with active participation of the care organisations "Thuiszorg Westelijke Mijnstreek" and "Zorggroep Noord-Limburg" and the health insurance agencies "Zorgkantoor Zuid-Limburg" and "Zorgkantoor Noord-en Midden Limburg."

References

[1] Willems Ch.G. and Vlieger S. de. The use of ICT in the delivery of unplannable care. In: Assistive Technology from virtuality to reality A.Pruski and H.Knops eds. IOS press Amsterdam 2005 pp 188-193

[2] Arnaert A. Tele-nursing for the elderly- The case of videotelephony care: an explorative study Thesis Katholic University of Leuven 2001
[3] Sanford J.A. Jones M.Daviou O, Grogg K, Butterfield T. Using telerehabilitation to identify home modification needs Assistive Technology. 2004 Summer; 16(1):43-53
[4] Iwabuchi M, Nakamura K, Alm N, Sakai S, Abe S A cell phone-based Electronic personal Profiler for care and support information. In: Assistive Technology : From Virtuality to Reality, Pruski A, Knops H (eds) IOS press Amsterdam 2005
[5] Vlaskamp, F., Cremers, G., en Willems, Ch., Zorgarrangementen voor specifieke cliëntgroepen in de thuiszorg, rapport in het kader van het project ICT Onplanbare, Zorg, Hoensbroek: iRv, maart 2004.
[6] The technology involved with videotelephony and monitoring behavior was delivered by Qou Vadis Nederland BV a, system integrator in the project.
[7] Thuiszorg Westelijke Mijnstreek Sittard Geleen and Zorggroep Noord Limburg Tegelen participated.
[8] Guillen S, Arredondo MT, Traver, Garcia JM, Fernandez C. Multimedia telehomecare system using a standard TV set IEEE trans Biomed Eng 2002 49: 1431-1437
[9] Herbert M.A., Korabek B. Stakeholder readiness for telehomecare: implications for implementation Telemed J.E.Health 2004 10: 85-92

Promoting Independence for Older Persons with Disabilities
W.C. Mann and A. Helal (Eds.)
IOS Press, 2006

Tele-Home Care / Care Coordination in the Rural Environment

Sydney WERTENBERGER[a,1]
[a]*John J. Pershing VA Medical Center, Poplar Bluff, MO USA*

Abstract. As a small rural VA Medical Center, we have embraced the challenges of providing high quality, accessible health care. Utilizing a business planning process with strong clinical leadership, we developed and implemented a successful home-telehealth program whose patients' profile includes advanced age, chronic disease processes and the desire to remain independent. The challenges of the rural environment provided opportunities for creative programming. Collaboration between technology, staff and patients have had statistically positive results for our patients and Medical Center.

Keywords. Telehealth, rural health care, care coordination

Introduction

The John J. Pershing Veteran's administration Medical Center is a small, very rural medical center located in southeast Missouri, approximately 160 miles south of Saint Louis, Mo. The medical center provides full service primary care for approximately 18,000 veterans, the majority of whom are male over the age of 65 and with multiple chronic health care problems. Services offered at the medical center include: in-patient acute care, active out-patient treatment for primary care and mental health services, telemedicine services and multiple out patient specialty clinics, and a nursing home care unit. The medical center has five full service primary care community based clinics, which are located between 76 and 126 miles from the medical center. These community based out-patient clinics (CBOC's) also offer mental health services. The very rural setting of this health care environment offers unique challenges and opportunities in health care planning program/development and implementation. The challenges include but are not limited to: access to care, health care costs and efficiencies, patient and staff transportation /travel, limited community resources, limited communication systems, and multiple geographic/regional issues which impact patients and the health care systems that serve them. Additionally, rural environments have limited health care options and shortages of health care providers.

Approximately 20 to 25 % of all Americans live in a rural environment on approximately 80% of the United States land mass. Generally rural communities tend to have a larger percentage of elderly patients, and they are likely to be poorer in health and economic status [1]. The rural areas have fewer health care providers, medical resources, such as hospitals. Rural communities are also characterized by a high rate of chronic illnesses such as hypertension, cardiovascular disease, obstructive lung disease and diabetes. Rural communities also have their own culture, which emphasizes independence and self-reliance as a community value [2]. Often professionals not from within the community are viewed as "outsiders". The " lack of trust " between "outside" providers and the patients is reflected in diminished follow through related to the need for specialty care referrals outside the community, as well as diminished compliance with patient education…" [3]

The unique geographic issues of a rural environment (such as terrain, isolation, geographic distance between points of access to care and weather), combined with the unique culture of the patients in our communities, has facilitated careful, innovative strategic planning combined with sound business planning, in order to meet the needs of the patients we serve. Our patient population reflects that: 85% of adults age 65 and older have at least one chronic disease and over 62% have two or more chronic diseases (4). The need to be efficient and cost effective in the current health care economy is a significant concern. Care of patients with chronic illnesses consumes over 70% of the United States health care budget annually [4]. The business planning process utilized is not unique to a tele-home care program, but rather to all new clinical endeavors within the Medical Center. The business process utilized includes: a description of the business: how does it integrate into/with our existing system of care, why is this financially effective: reviewing the traditional financial indicators, as well as the potential value to the organization, identification of potential negligence/high risk concerns, resources required including personnel, space and equipment, marketing plans and anticipated outcomes. Two sections of the business planning process received the primary focus of the interdisciplinary planning and later implementation work group's time and attention: a clear well communicated description of the business, and a cost analysis that demonstrated not only the dollar cost, but carefully reviewed the value of home telehealth for our patient population, and health care community.

We also reviewed the health care planning literature to ensure that our actions were consistent with experts in the field of health care planning. This included the Institute of Medicines (IOM) 2001 report "Crossing the Quality Chasm" [5]. This report emphasized the need to reform the healthcare system fueled by the increasing numbers of patients with chronic illnesses and the consumer driven identified need of care that is " customized according to the patients' needs and values, evidenced based, the patient is the source of control, needs are anticipated waste is decreased, knowledge flows freely, and …." [5]. The need to ensure appropriate care of patients with chronic diseases, working with them collaboratively to develop treatment goals and objectives is a central theme in the literature [5]. Concomitantly our nursing staff, community health staff and other members of the health care team attended several off station workshops and presentations related to these topics.

In the planning process it was noted that patients for a new tele-home care program might be referred from multiple points of care within the organization. We had multiple patients who accessed the emergency room, and or urgent care clinics for treatment of acute symptoms for chronic conditions, which if closely monitored and treated promptly might never need urgent care or emergency room visits. This phenomenon is reflective of national norms within the United States, where emergency room visits have increased 14% between 1992 and 1999 [3]. As a result of this information integrated through the development of our business plan, in response to our goals and objectives of providing appropriate access to care, managing patients with chronic illness so that they could safely have the independence and quality of life they want, and our need to have sounds financial plans, we opted for development of a tele-home care program, consistent the Department of Veterans Affairs Care Coordination/Home tele-health Program.

VHA has defined care coordination in two ways, from the professional view point and from the patients view point. The professional definition of Care Coordination is " the wider application of care and case management principles to the delivery of health services using health informatics, disease management and Telehealth technologies to facilitate access to care and improve the health of designated individuals and populations with the specific intent of providing the right care at right place at the right time" [6]. The patients definition of care coordination is "the use of new information technologies that connect people to health services that help ensure the right care happens in the right place at the right time" [6]. These definitions were consistent with the stated goals and objectives in our strategic planning process, and with our literature review. This approach offered us a way to provide close frequent monitoring of patients with chronic health conditions, so that prompt intervention could be provided. Prompt intervention had the potential to minimized complications from, or acute exacerbations of chronic diseases. This program also provided a viable opportunity to assist our patients to remain at home, and as independent as possible. It furthered the concept of the patient as an active partner in his/her own health care. It appeared to offer cost savings through cost avoidance by: having the patient cared for at the appropriate level of care (complexity), thereby decreasing the use of resource intensive levels of care such as the emergency room/urgent care, and in-patient hospital admissions. It was projected that tele-home care/care coordination program would not only improve access to care for the patients who participated but that these actions might decompress our urgent care areas, and allow these resources to be more easily accessed by those who needed them.

1. Actions/Implementation

We did not have the funds necessary to develop and implement this program. Therefore, we wrote an access to care grant request identifying how the implementation of a care coordination/home tele-health program would assist us in caring for our chronic disease patients, and identifying potential cost avoidance/cost savings this program would generate. We received an initial seed money grant, which we utilized to purchase equipment. We chose to make our initial purchases the most complex tele-home care equipment. We postulated that the initial success of the program would be based on good communication with the primary care teams, and tangible success from the monitoring of clinical and financial program outcomes. Developing and implementing a home tele-health program in a rural environment has some technical issues and barriers including distance and multiple different communication/telephone systems from one rural community to another (our service area covers hundreds of square miles). Additionally staff and patients need to be familiar with the equipment, competent and comfortable with its use as well as know how and when to access support, often from distant sites.

We consulted with others who had utilized this technology, ordered our equipment, identified staff that had the "right" background for a program such as this. The equipment ordered had been utilized elsewhere within the VHA system, with positive outcomes. We identified that for a care coordinator we needed clinical expertise in patient assessment/reassessment, case management experience, good patient educator skills, competence with care of chronic disease patients and the abilities to assist with patients becoming active partners in their own health care (patient self-management skills) Staff selected for working with this program included Advance practice nurses, and Masters prepared social workers. Assignments of care coordinators to patients was based on the patients' identified need/treatment goals that were developed jointly with the primary care team, patient and the care coordinators. We identified that we needed strong collaboration between the clinical and technology staff. Therefore we developed and placed the telemedicine coordinator position aligned organizationally within the care coordination/home tele–health staff. It became apparent as we went through the process of developing this program that staff and patients need to develop trust and understanding with each other and the technology tools. We anticipated that education and dependable support, combined with clinical and administrative champions/program advocates, and medical center leadership encouragement central to program success.

Patient selection for initial referral to the program came from reviewing those patients with chronic diseases who frequently were seen in the urgent care/emergency room, or seen by their primary care clinic teams more than once every four months. Education for the medical center medical staff (all providers), primary care clinic teams, and the urgent care/emergency room personnel regarding this new program was also provided. We aligned out care coordination/home tele-health program organizationally with our community health nursing program, emphasizing that it is another resource at maintaining the patient within his/her own home. Professional reference material for staff and marketing literature for patients including success stories from others who had implemented care coordination/home-Telehealth programs were shared and left with/at possible referral sources/sites. In summary: we identified why we wanted to start this program, and made sure that leadership of the medical center was supportive of this initiative, that we had clinical and administrative champions identified, that we included all stake holders, that we educated staff, and patients and we formalized the program through the development policies/procedures, informed consent forms, position descriptions, identified staff competencies, and readily available references to keep staff on track with new processes. Additionally we brought in expert speakers on care coordination/home tele-health and sent staff to conferences on care coordination/home tele-health.

We also involved patients, developing tools to educate them about the program, and to make them informed consumers/partners in their own care. We helped patients make the link that programs such as these, utilizing technology as a tool, assisted the patient in remaining independent, and provided them with easy access to care. Patients were also provided opportunity to learn not only "survival" skills for living with a chronic disease(s), but were provided support and education to further build their own self management skills, fostering their informed independence.

To evaluate the programs effectiveness we had monitors/evaluation criteria for the program success. We had full program review after the first 12 months of the program. We did incremental "mini" program reviews prior to the end of the first year of the program, but utilized them to ensure that our program and process design were appropriate. We utilized the "mini" reviews to make program adjustments and as opportunities for improvement. As with all new programs that involved change, and people, frequent positive reinforcement and review facilitated the changes. The business functions were addressed by staff with expertise in that area. These functions were considered very necessary if the new program would remain viable.

2. Outcomes

The first annual program review of our care coordination/home tele-health program was completed in August of 2005. A closed record review was performed on all patients who had been in the program for one year. The following outcomes for patients in our care coordination/home tele-health program were identified: 1.) Scheduled primary care visits decreased by 20.2% 2.) Unscheduled primary care visits (clinic walk-ins) decreased by 25% 3.) Nursing only visits to primary care decreased by 83% 4.)Urgent care/emergency room visits decreased by 53% 5.)Appintment "no shows" decreased by 53% 6.) In-patient admissions for these patients decreased by 42%. Additional information gathered during this review included: no patient complaints regarding this program were reported to the patient advocate, or supervisory personnel. No equipment had been "lost" or destroyed during the year. There had been no staff turnover during the year. The most frequent diagnosis for the patients enrolled in the program included: chronic obstructive airway disease, congestive heart failure, diabetes, and hypertension.

These statistics demonstrates that this program was very effective in providing patients the opportunity to have prompt access to care at the appropriate level of acuity, with patient and staff satisfaction and cost avoidance. All of the equipment purchased has paid for itself in less than one year.

References

[1] USDA National Agriculture Library Rural Information Center, http://www.nal.usda.gov/ric/ricpubs/what_is_rural.htm. Retrieved November 15, 2005.

[2] "Assess Your Towns People, One of the Elements of Rural Culture". http://kansassampler.org/wekan/people.html. Retrieved November 15, 2005.

[3] Baldwin, Sisk, Watts, McCubbin, Brocksmidt, Marion, 1998.

[4] Cherry, D.D., Curt C.W., & Woodwell, D.A. (2003). National Ambulatory Medical Care Survey: 2001 Summary. CDC Advance Data from Vital and Health Statistics.

[5] Institute of Medicine. 2001. Crossing the Quality Chasm: A new health system for the 21st Century. Executive Summary. Washington, DC: National Academies Press

[6] VHA Office of Telemedicine and Care Coordination, http://www.va.gov/occ/ Retrieved November 15, 2005.

Promoting Independence for Older Persons with Disabilities
W.C. Mann and A. Helal (Eds.)
IOS Press, 2006

e-Health Innovations: Internet-Base Caregiver Education and Support

Jeff LOOMIS[a,1], Magaly FREYTES[a], and Megan WITTE[a]
[a]*UF Center for Telehealth, University of Florida, Gainesville, FL USA*

Abstract. The UF Center for Telehealth's AlzOnline project provides Internet and telephone-based support, information, and skills training to caregivers of persons with progressive dementia. Since its inception, AlzOnline has worked through community service leaders to provide caregivers of persons with progressive dementia, looking for relief in the day-to-day tasks of caregiving providing education and support. In year 2004 and 2005, AlzOnline had over 240,000 visits to its web-based services.

Keywords. Telehealth, e-health, caregiver, alzheimer's disease

Introduction

Approximately 4.5 million people in the U.S. over the age of 60 have Alzheimer's disease or a closely related form of progressive dementia. The economic consequences of these disorders are substantial, costing the nation $100 billion a year in direct and indirect medical care, lost productivity, and care [1]. s one of the leading states with the highest incidence of Alzheimer's disease the impact of Alzheimer's disease is felt strongly in Florida [4]. More than 435,000 Floridians currently have some form of mild to severe dementia [3]. Statistics estimate that family or friends are caring for 75 percent of persons with mild to severe dementia in the home [2]. As the nation's healthcare system faces enormous funding challenges, innovative programs that provide resources at lower cost must be sought.

One promising tool available to healthcare consumers is the ability to gather health information, education, and support through the use of the World Wide Web. In 2003, the Pew Internet Foundation reported that approximately 93 million adults have searched the Internet for some form of health information. Of these adult Internet users, 73 percent reported an improvement in health information and services [6]. A 2004 report from the National Alliance for Caregiving and the Alzheimer's Association reported that despite the availability of local support services designed to offer caregivers with a variety of education and support services, less than ten percent of Alzheimer's caregivers participate in these traditional support group services for help or information. Thirty-one percent of the 227 Alzheimer's caregivers surveyed actually access support and information though the Internet [2].

Though the Internet holds considerable promise for helping health consumers, the true measure of a good health care model is its accessibility, quality of the services provided, and the ability to deliver services in a cost effective manner. The purpose of this paper is to present an evaluation of Alzheimer's Caregiver Support Online (AlzOnline), an Internet-based caregiver support network for caregivers of elders with progressive dementia. The specific objectives of this paper are to look at the consumer satisfaction data and determine if AlzOnline is an effective health model based on accessibility, quality, and cost.

1. Background

AlzOnline is an Internet and telephone based education and support service for caregivers of elders with Alzheimer's disease and other progressive dementias. It was established by the State of Florida Department of Elder Affairs and the University of Florida's Center for Telehealth. The program's goal is to fill the gap that exists between caregivers' needs and the resources available to help them look after a family member with Alzheimer's disease. AlzOnline utilizes a team-based approach of several health practitioners, including occupational therapists (OTs), a pharmacist, and a mental health counselor. The specific objectives of the AlzOnline project are to, (1) provide Internet-based information, education and support for caregivers of individuals with progressive dementia, (2) serve as a statewide resource and clearinghouse for statewide services, and (3) provide a toll-free telephone line to ensure easy and rapid access to information and support about dementia caregiving issues.

AlzOnline is geared toward relieving caregiver stress and providing practical tips on managing the difficulties of caregiving. It is an interactive program where caregivers can visit and participate in caregiver education, support classes, and an active message board. AlzOnline also provides information on the latest developments in dementia research and strategies for increasing caregiver and care recipient quality of life to support aging in place. A Spanish version of the program is also available.

Research shows that practical information regarding activities of daily living (ADLs) for caregivers of elders with Alzheimer's disease is limited. Findings from a recent national survey conducted by the National Alliance for Caregiving (2004) found that 62 percent of caregivers provide assistance with at least one ADL, while 36 percent provide assistance with three or more ADLs [5]. AlzOnline recently expanded its services with practical, ready to use information regarding ADLs under the direction of the University of Florida, Department of Occupational Therapy. The information presented on the site is in Power Point form and includes toileting, dressing, bathing, grooming, and eating, all given through the expertise of an OT. All presentations include a variety of pictures, with references to websites where products and adaptive equipment discussed may be purchased. A separate "Tips and Techniques" page is available for caregivers to print out as a quick reference. Each presentation ends with a survey for the caregiver to complete to determine how the information was perceived, and what improvements could be added to make the presentations more user- friendly and practical. Caregivers are also encouraged to ask questions and post them on the AlzOnline message board. OTs are also on-hand to provide specific assistance to e-mails and phone calls received by the project coordinator.

Another problem commonly reported by families and caregivers, is the management of medications. It is estimated that 73 percent of persons with Alzheimer's need assistance managing their medications [2]. As part of the expanded services, a series of classes intended to provide information, suggestions and practical solutions to the most common problems associated with medication use were developed under the supervision of the University of Florida College of Pharmacy. Following the format of the ADL classes, the medication management classes were also developed using a Power Point format, and included information on giving medicines as prescribed, communicating with the physician, overview of medicines that should be used with caution, and a Personal Medication Record (or PMR) was developed to help caregivers keep track of the medications the person they caring for are taking.

AlzOnline is designed to meet their specific objectives by offering the following services, (1) *Caregiving Topics* offering a variety of written and audio recordings on healthcare topics specific to caregiving for a person with progressive dementia, (2) *Classroom* designed to address specific caregiver challenges, such as managing medications, activities of daily living, caregiver training and stress management, (3) caregiver-led *Message Board,* an interactive virtual support group where caregivers can receive peer support and advice. The message board is monitored by the AlzOnline team to dispel any myths that may arise, and also provide supplemental caregiving information. Links to local and national resources (Area Agencies on Aging, State-sponsored Memory Disorder Clinics, National Eldercare Locator) are also available through the website.

Since its inception in August 2000, Alzheimer's Caregiver Support Online has, established an extensive network of Internet-based education and support services for caregivers of individuals with progressive dementia, hosted telephone-based professional presentations for caregivers on a variety of relevant topics, and developed a Spanish language version of AlzOnline. The AlzOnline team works with community leaders in the Hispanic / Latino community to raise awareness of Alzheimer's disease, creating culturally sensitive educational material, and integrating the online and telephone-based services into the community.

For AlzOnline to have a statewide and national impact on assisting informal caregivers, the services provided by AlzOnline must be easy to access, and must also provide a quality service. In addition, we must attract more caregivers to our service in a cost efficient manner.

2. Method

To evaluate our program, access, quality, and cost efficiency were formally assessed.

Access: To determine our success with regard to access we collected traffic data between July 1, 2003 and June 30, 2005. To track the number of visits to the website we measured traffic by total visits and unique visits. A visit is defined as any action initiated when a visitor views it first page. A unique visit is identified by IP address a session cookie, only counting a visit in a 30-day period.

Quality: Between July 1, 2003 and June 30, 2005 we used the online satisfaction survey to measure quality. Throughout the website visitors are given an opportunity to complete a satisfaction survey. We also send persons who have accessed our service via e-mail a follow-up message asking them to evaluate our service, directing them to the online survey. Data gathered from this survey is used to evaluate our program, and this feedback is used to improve our product.

Cost Effectiveness: The State of Florida provides reimbursement through the Area Agencies on Aging to contract agencies to provide support group services through the National Family Caregiver Support Program. The program offers family caregivers local support group services in their local community, and is normally accessed on a monthly basis. To compare the cost of face-to-face support services with that of the

AlzOnline education and support services, we took the average of the current state reimbursement rate under the National Family Caregiver Support Program, and compared this with services accessed through AlzOnline. This was done because even though many caregivers will come back more than one time, a unique visit was a closer representation of face-to-face services accessed through the National Family Caregiver Support Program.

3. Results

Access: During year 2003-2005, AlzOnline averaged approximately 247,298 visits, serving 94,298 unique visitors. This number of visitors to AlzOnline has grown significantly each year (Figure 1). As more research is done on the benefit of caregiver interventions, AlzOnline is positioned to continue bringing the latest in caregiver interventions to caregivers.

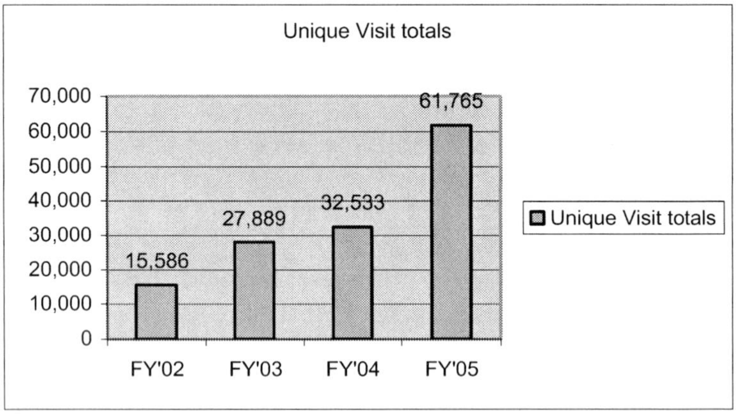

Figure 1. Total unique visits annually

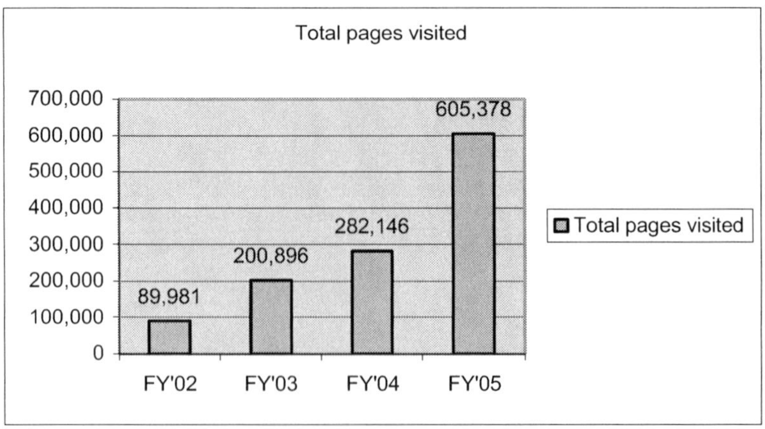

Figure 2. Total pages visited annually

The monthly average of services delivered:

- 3,929 unique visits
- Over 10,000 total visits
- 1000 visits to the Message Board
- 220 visits to the pre-recorded educational material

Quality: AlzOnline measured quality of services through a six-question online satisfaction survey. (N=162) Through the survey, caregivers were able to rate their ease of navigation through the website, the information, and educational services, and offer feedback on how services impact them as caregivers. Feedback was also reviewed on a monthly basis and the recommendations were implemented as necessary.

Table 1. Did you find our site easy to navigate?

User Responses	Count (N=162)	Percentage
No Answer	4	2.47%
Very easy to navigate	108	66.67%
Somewhat easy to navigate	46	28.40%
Somewhat difficult to navigate	4	2.47%
Very difficult to navigate	0	0.00%

Table 2. Overall, how satisfied are you with our services?

User Responses	Count (N=162)	Percentage
No Answer	16	9.88%
Very satisfied	106	65.67%
Somewhat satisfied	33	20.37%
Somewhat dissatisfied	5	3.09%
Very dissatisfied	2	1.23%

Table 3. How much has AlzOnline helped you in your role as a caregiver?

User Responses	Count (N=162)	Percentage
No Answer	31	19.14%
It helped a lot	84	51.85%
It helped a little	41	25.31%
It has not helped	6	3.70%
It has made things worse	0	0.00%

Table 4. How has AlzOnline helped you as a caregiver?

User Responses	Count (N=162)	Percentage
No Answer	87	53.70%
Site provided resources & information	30	18.52%
Site provided support	17	10.49%
Provided information and support	22	13.58%
No change	1	0.62%
Other	5	3.09%

Representative responses: "This has given me new hope in a desperate situation, these services are crucial for people dealing with this disease and I hope more places can be offered so that people with Alzheimer's do not have to suffer alone with this horrifying disease." "They provide information that I can use daily for caregiving. The message boards let me see what others are experiencing with the disease and it is there if I should need to vent."

Table 5a. Will you revisit AlzOnline in the future?

User Responses	Count (N=162)	Percentage
No Answer	7	4.32%
Yes	151	93.21%
No	1	0.62%
Undecided	3	1.85%

Table 5b. If you will not visit AlzOnline again, please tell us why not.

User Responses	Count (N=162)	Percentage
No Answer	162	100%

Table 6. Please provide us with any additional comments or suggestions

(Anecdotal answers given)
Many of the responses received, were from caregivers offering their gratitude for the services received through AlzOnline. A few responses offered feedback on how we could improve the site.

Overall, those caregivers responding to the satisfaction survey were all generally satisfied with the services provided.

Cost Effectiveness: Currently the State of Florida provides reimbursement through community services agencies providing support group services through the Family Caregiver Support Program. This program offers family caregivers local support group services in their local community. Between 2003 and 2004 services provided through these support group services (n=5) were reimbursed at approximately $23.30/hr, and this figure did not include respite reimbursement, which averages to $16.40/hr. AlzOnline provides support services through an active peer support message board that acts as a virtual support group, pre-recorded classroom material, and a toll-free telephone line. Based on the number of unique visitors averages from 2003-2004, web services were delivered at a cost of $2.34 per individual visit, or $7.68 per unique visitor. Because many support groups offer their services on a monthly basis, we consider the number of unique visits as the better comparison with face-to-face support groups however, a person with a computer can access AlzOnline at any time of the day making this a very cost effective way of obtaining support when and where needed.

4. Limitations

Web-based services offer their own set of challenges. In the area of measuring visits, we have relied on counting unique visits, as a measure of success. Web hosting companies as a standard practice only audit unique visits in a 30-day window. With health seekers becoming more aware of Internet attacks, the removal of Internet cookies can account for a visitor being counted more than one time. With a dial-up connection a visitor can also have more than one IP address, and be counted more than once. With regard to quality, we are not able to always obtain visitor feedback through the satisfaction survey. Although everyone has an equal opportunity to complete a survey, we may not be receiving feedback from health seekers who may not have had their needs met. In addition, another limitation associated with quality measures is the brief and generic nature of the survey. Finally, in the area of cost efficiency, there are 13 Area Agencies on Aging providing support through the National Family Caregiver Support Program; we were only able to gather data from 5 of the 13 service providers.

5. Conclusion

The AlzOnline project reaches informal caregivers of elders with progressive dementia who may not necessarily be able to attend local support group services due to issues such as lack of transportation or not having someone to stay with their loved one. AlzOnline has proven itself to be a quality program that is accessible when and where health information, education, and support are needed. Services delivered through Internet technology can offer quality health information and support services at a fraction of the cost of traditional face-to-face services. The problem with telehealth or e-health programs is often lack sustainability once the funding stream is turned off. What is needed is a way to generate capital that will sustain AlzOnline and similar programs. To address this, AlzOnline will begin to develop and offer online classes for the professional caregiver. Because, the State of Florida requires professional organization caring for Alzheimer's patients to obtain initial dementia-specific training, the Internet offers an opportunity for AlzOnline to deliver formal education online as a potential revenue stream. In conclusion, access to Internet-based caregiver education and support will increase as the baby-boom generation begins to retire and age in place. Informal caregivers are an important part of the healthcare continuum. It is imperative that we consider innovative services such as AlzOnline to assist the informal caregi ver.

Acknowledgements

The State of Florida Department of Elder Affairs, and the University of Florida College of Public Health and Health Professions sponsor this project.

References

[1] Alzheimer's Association. (2005, May 15). About Alzheimer's disease statistics. Retrieved September 30, 2005 from http://alz.org/Resources/FactSheets/FSAlzheimerStats.pdf

[2] Alzheimer's Association & National Alliance for Caregiving (n.d.) Families care: Alzheimer's caregiving in the United Stets 2004. Retrieved September 30, 2005 from http://www.alz.org/Resources/FactSheets/Caregiverreport.pdf

[3] Florida Department of Elder Affairs. (n.d.) Florida County Profiles 2004. Retrieved September 30, 2005 from http://elderaffairs.state.fl.us/english/Stats/DOCS/2004cp.pdf

[4] Hebert, L. E., Scherr, P. A., Bienias, J. L., Bennett, D. A., & Evans, D. A.. (2004). State-specific projections through 2025 of Alzheimer's disease prevalence [Electronic version]. Neurology, 62, 1654.

[5] National Alliance for Caregiving & AARP. (2004). Caregiving in the U.S.. Retrieved September 30, 2005 from http://www.caregiving.org/data/04finalreport.pdf

[6] Pew Internet & American Life Project. (2003, July 16). Internet health resources. Retrieved September 30, 2005 from http://www.pewinternet.org/pdfs/PIP_Health_Report_July_2003.pdf

Promoting Independence for Older Persons with Disabilities
W.C. Mann and A. Helal (Eds.)
IOS Press, 2006

Ethical Considerations of Home Monitoring Technology

Janice BLANCHARD[a]
[a] *Society of Certified Senior Advisors*

Abstract. Telehealth applications are being developed and marketed to meet the challenges of an aging society. Preliminary research into viability, however, has concentrated predominately on cost effectiveness and technological efficiency; moral, legal, and ethical issues remain largely unaddressed in research, evaluation, and practice. This panel discussion examines such issues as privacy, confidentiality, paternalism, equity of access and the role of government and marketplace in shaping the future of this emerging field.

Keywords. Telehealth, ethics, home monitoring

Introduction

Innovators and leaders from a variety of fields - computer technology, gerontology, medicine, and academia - to name a few, have collaborated in recent years to form a new sub-specialty: Home monitoring technology (also referred to as home health technology and home-based telemedicine). Under the larger umbrella of telemedicine, home monitoring technology consists of a variety of products, systems, and services (many of which are still under development) to aid disabled and senior populations, particularly the cognitively impaired, with every day tasks; health monitoring; early detection of diseases; and detecting and emergency response situations [2].

Home monitoring technology and other home-based telemedicine programs are emerging in response to several external forces: A need to contain spiraling health care costs, a growing population of chronically ill and frail elders, public policies and consumer demands that support aging in place initiatives, and private companies that recognize the market potential of 77 million graying baby boomers [1, 2]. Until recently, monitoring technology has existed only in research settings; however cheaper, more readily available digital technology means that relatively affordable systems will become increasingly available over the next few years.

Preliminary research into the viability of home monitoring technology has concentrated predominately on cost effectiveness and technological efficiency; moral and ethical issues remain largely unaddressed in research, evaluation, and practice [1]. This paper explores some of these ethical considerations as they pertain to home monitoring technology and elder clients.

1. From Simple to Complex Systems

The goal of home monitoring technology is to enhance the ability of disabled and older adults to age in place (i.e., to live independently in their homes as long as possible), while at the same time lowering long-term care costs, and easing caregiver burden [2]. Home monitoring technology ranges from simple, stand-alone devices to complex, integrated systems.

At the low-technology end are unidirectional communication devices such as the personal emergency response system (PERS), a wearable, lightweight, waterproof necklace or wristband that is activated by pressing a button, which sends a signal via telephone line to a response center. A trained technician at the center determines the severity of the situation and takes appropriate action.

At the moderate-technology level, motion detection sensors track an elder's movement within the home. These low-cost sensors are typically wired to a communications device that transmits the data over the Internet to a processing station, notifying someone if the data meets certain criteria. Also found at the moderate-technology level are home health monitoring systems connecting seniors via phone lines or the Internet to health providers in order to monitor and analyze patient's vital signs, symptoms, behavior, and/or health knowledge.

At the high-technology end, elaborate systems are evolving, such as the one described below by Intel Corporation.

> *Its [Intel's] research goes beyond motion detectors and pillbox sensors to include things like pressure sensors on an Alzheimer's patient's favorite chair, networks of cameras, and tiny radio tags embedded in household items and clothing that communicate with tag readers in floor mats, shelves, and walls. From the pattern of these signals, a computer can deduce what a person is doing and intervene—giving instructions over a networked television or bedside radio, or wirelessly alerting a caregiver* [5].

2. Every Picture Tells A Story

Moderate- and high-tech home monitoring can implicitly (through sensors and radio tags) and explicitly (through cameras and microphones) record details of a person's life from the mundane to the highly personal. How much did someone toss and turn in bed? How much time did a person spend in the bathroom? How many visitors (and who were they) stopped by during the course of the day? By either method, a "picture" emerges of a person's daily life, and the collection and use of that is the crux of the technology. The routines and locations being monitored, the destination of the information, and under what circumstances the information is given varies between systems and situations, as illustrated in the following examples:

1. An 85-year-old woman with osteoporosis is monitored 24/7 throughout her home by sensors that check for signs that she has fallen. The information is sent via a wireless network to a home health monitoring facility, which adheres to a confidentiality agreement disclosing information only to a nearby daughter, and only when a fall or other emergency has been detected.

2. A 67-year-old man with coronary heart disease and sleep apnea is monitored for three nights via a phone device as he sleeps. The information is sent to a diagnostic testing facility, where a report is run and delivered to his physician.
3. A 71-year-old man living alone with early onset dementia is monitored 24/7 throughout his house by a combination of sensor and video monitoring. The information is sent via wireless to a secure Web site where his son can check on him throughout the day. Pre-set triggers (e.g., smoke alarm, door bell, door alarm) can alert his son or emergency personnel with a phone call or email.

Regardless of how or why people are monitored at home, the rationale generally remains the same – to reduce the risk of adverse health outcomes and to provide reassurance to the elders, as well as family, friends, or health providers that someone is watching out for them.

3. The Devil is in the Details

So, what could be ethically troubling about ensuring our elders' safety, enhancing their ability to live independently in their own homes, and providing reassurance to them and their loved ones that if trouble arises, someone will be there to answer the call? The devil is in the details.

It has been stated or can be inferred that moderate and high-end home monitoring technology systems are based on the following assumptions:

1. People prefer to age in place in their own homes, and home monitoring systems significantly increase their ability to do so.
2. A person's right to privacy is second to the need for safety and security, and individuals are willing to make this trade-off.
3. Safety and security can be enhanced through careful observation of images or data by detecting adverse events before they happen and responding more quickly when they do occur.
4. Another person or form of technology is willing, capable, and reliable at monitoring images or data and drawing the appropriate conclusion to act or not act.
5. Images and data collected would be used only for the purposes of enhancing safety and security, and to inform or reassure the care recipient and selected others.
6. Home monitoring technology will lower health care costs.
7. Home monitoring technology will ease caregiver burden.

Each of these assumptions pose a number of concerns that need to be considered, regardless of who we are monitoring or for what purposes. This is not to say monitoring technology is inherently bad or ineffective; it does mean that we want to support a system that is ethically guided and philosophically sound. We will only examine the assumptions regarding privacy in this article. Examples of some of the ethical issues raised by the other assumptions are illustrated in Table 1.

4. The Crossroads of Privacy and Safety

Surprisingly, the "right to privacy" is not spelled out in the U.S. Constitution. However, the U.S. Supreme Court has repeatedly upheld that privacy is an implied right in several of the amendments in the Bill of Rights. Many of the court cases in which the right to privacy has been upheld have been related to personal/private health decisions (e.g., Griswold v. Connecticut and Roe v. Wade). Likewise, our right to privacy in health matters has also been protected by legislation, the most recent being the 1996 Health Insurance Portability and Accountability Act (HIPAA) that went into effect early in 2003.

Where the right to privacy intersects with safety and security is less clear, particularly with regard to health matters. For example, adults have the right to smoke tobacco and drink alcohol, although both are associated with negative health outcomes -the right to make a personal (private) choice is given precedent over safety. Contrarily, one is not legally supported in making such choices with regard to illicit drugs or wearing a seatbelt - personal safety is held as the higher standard.

The right to privacy versus safety and security is a complex ethical issue that is playing out in an increasing number of arenas. For example, many Americans believe that it is not only a parental duty, but their parental *right* to closely monitor their children's online activities – placing safety and security over their child's right to privacy. What constitutes "close monitoring", however, varies widely between households, from talking to a child about their online activities, to keeping the computer in the main living area, to using software that tracks online chats, Web navigation, and emails.

In the field of aging, the issues of privacy versus safety and security have also been debated. For example, the installation of electronic monitoring devices or "granny cams" has been hotly contested between various stakeholders. In particular, family members often wish for such devices in long-term care facilities to protect their loved one from harm or neglect, while those facilities have argued that such devices violate an elder's right to privacy, as well as that of the facility's staff. To date, several states, including Florida and Maryland, have pilot projects to study the effects of granny cams, but only Texas has legislation specifically allowing them in residents' rooms.

Privacy issues are multi-faceted in home monitoring. Simply defining the concept presents a complex task. For example, if one defines it as the ability to control access over what we share with another, the ability to maintain privacy in a monitored home is tenuous -- one cannot simultaneously be under real-time observation and still maintain the ability to decide what will be shared. Therefore, if a home is fully wired, can one have any reasonable expectation for privacy?

Beyond privacy of the person, lie privacy concerns regarding collected data. Currently there are no standard protocols for protecting the security of email, telemetry and electronic health records. Further, firewalls and encryption, while they may slow down the process, are unlikely to deter someone motivated to access personal health records [3]. Wireless transmissions pose even greater concerns [1]. Concerns regarding privacy, confidentiality, and security of health information have always existed; however, the ease, extent and context in which they may be breached are intensified with the electronic exchange of information [1].

Whether elders, particularly baby boomers, will be willing to trade privacy for security and safety has not yet been firmly established.

5. Conclusion

Demographic, economic, and healthcare trends portend a long-term care disaster in the coming decades if we do not aggressively pursue a strategy to meet the long-term care needs of Americans. To this end, many are looking to information technology and telemedicine to provide some solutions. Cheaper, faster, and more efficient digital technology has catapulted telemedicine into the 21st century: Telemedicine has grown from 4 active programs in 1990 [6] to over 360 programs in 2001 in the U.S. [4]. In financial terms, the U.S. federal government spent nearly $1 billion on telemedicine research, grants, and other funding in 2002 alone [6].

The adoption of health technology is often driven by cost effectiveness and overall efficiency, with little regard given to its ethical appropriateness and justification [1]. We critically need a moral and ethical framework for home-based telemedicine to provide the best chance of consumer adoption and satisfaction, improvements in quality of care and quality of life, protection of personal privacy and autonomy.

It is at the birth of a technology, the opening of a new era when we must most intently look past it to the future. We must parallel the development of new technology with the evolution of ethical responsibility and intelligence to control it. We must match the ability to collect information with the legislation and prudence to manage it. And we must protect our personal rights as strongly as we wish to protect our personal health.

Table 1. Examples of ethical issues raised by home monitoring technology in an aging population:

1. **Privacy of information.** Who has access to data and how it will be used? Can it be bought and sold? How will privacy, confidentiality, and security of user information be assured?
2. **Privacy of person/place.** Can user control monitoring system (e.g., turn it off and on, or establish a monitor-free zone)? How is the privacy of others in the home maintained?
3. **Informed consent.** What constitutes informed consent, particularly with a technologically naïve or cognitively impaired person?
4. **Equity of access.** How do we develop equal access when technology use presupposes some technological sophistication, skills, and basic comfort level? Who will pay for services? Will it develop into a two-tier system of medical service delivery?
5. **Autonomy versus dependence.** Does home monitoring foster autonomy or dependence? What will be the consequences of perceived non-compliance?
6. **Paternalism.** Does the desire to "keep a better watch" over aging parents actually reveal or underscore a paternalistic attitude on the part of service providers, adult children, and/or the medical establishment towards elders?
7. **Patient and provider relationship.** What is the overall effect on quality of care? How are empathy, compassion and trust maintained via telecommunication?
8. **Medicalization of home.** Will long term monitoring change the character of home? How do we maintain the separation of public and private sphere?

References:

[1] Bauer, KA (2002). Home-based telemedicine: A survey of ethical issues. Cambridge Quarterly of Healthcare Ethics, 10, 137-146.

[2] CAST [Center for Aging Services Technology] (2003). Progress and possibilities: State of technology and aging services. White paper.

[3] Grigsby, J and Sanders, JH (1998). Telemedicine: Where it is and where it's going. *Annals of Internal Medicine*, 129:123-127.

[4] Hersh, WR, Helfand, M, Wallace, J, et al. (2001). Clinical outcomes resulting from telemedicine interventions: A systematic review. *BMC Medical Informatics and Decision Making* 1(5). Retrieved September 29, 2003, from http://www.biomedcentral.com/1472-6947/1/5

[5] Huang, GT (2003). Monitoring mom. As population matures, so do assisted-living technologies. MIT Technology Review, July/August.

[6] Whitten, P & Kuwahara, E (2003). Telemedicine from the payor perspective: Considerations for reimbursement decisions. *Disease Management Health Outcomes*, 11(5): 291-298.

Promoting Independence for Older Persons with Disabilities
W.C. Mann and A. Helal (Eds.)
IOS Press, 2006

How Family Caregivers of Persons with Alzheimer's Disease Obtain Online Resources

Jiaying SHEN [a]
[a] *Industrial and System Engineering Department, University of Wisconsin – Madison, Madison, Wi USA*

Abstract. This study is part of a larger project, exploring how to deploy the Internet as a tool to assist home care for people with Alzheimer's disease. This study followed a qualitative paradigm, investigating how the caregivers obtain online information resources for their regular online activities. The participants had four approaches to seek resources for their regular online activities and they usually started the information search with search engines like Yahoo or Google or with their preferred resources. The results provide a base in understanding caregivers' Internet behavior and provides guidance for improving Internet/web design and increasing use of websites.

Keywords. Internet, caregiving, alzheimer's disease

Introduction

Alzheimer's disease is common among the elderly. The prevalence of this disease among the population aged 85 and older is approximately 30 to 40% [3, 10, 23]. The number of Americans with Alzheimer's disease will grow to 11.3 million to 16 million by 2050 [14]. The family members of people with Alzheimer's disease play a fundamental role in the management of these pathologies. Eighty percent of the care provided to Alzheimer's patients in the community is provided by family members [21]. Caregiving could impact their physical and mental health, and expand their social network and activities [12, 13, 15, 19]. A report of Alzheimer's Association and the National Alliance for Caregiving shows that these caregivers provide the most difficult type of care, and are more exposed to the risk of physical strain and emotional stress compared to caregivers of other types of diseases.

The Internet can deliver health-related information and services; the Internet can also be an efficient means for delivering health risk assessments and health promotion modules [1, 16]. There is evidence that the Internet can be effective in enhancing patients and caregivers' social support and in promoting their emotional well-being and physical health [18]. For caregivers, the Internet has been used to deliver therapeutic interventions aimed at helping them to manage their anger, reduce their symptoms of depression and achieve positive developmental outcomes [24]. However, research that thoroughly and systematically examines the role computer or Internet - based technology can play in the care of persons with Alzheimer's disease is limited. A small number of studies have investigated the role of computer technology in caring for persons with Alzheimer disease.

ComputerLink is a computer system developed to assist caregivers of persons with Alzheimer's disease in providing home care. It consists of a communications module, information module and decision support module. It links caregivers to a nurse moderator and elevates the communication among caregivers [2]. The communication module permits several choices for public or private communication among caregivers: private mail, public bulletin board (forum) and Question and Answer segment (Q&A). In Forum, caregivers and the nurse moderator publicly post message for all users of ComputerLink; The Q&A section allows caregivers to post questions for response by a nurse moderator; Caregivers who desire private communication with other participant can choose the private mail option, which allows them to type in messages and send them directly to the desired recipients. The information module is an electronic encyclopedia, which provides over 200 indexed screens of information about Alzheimer's disease, caregiver issues, community resources for Alzheimer's disease and self-care for caregivers. The decisions support module assists caregivers in making choices consistent with their values using an analysis process that incorporates their own work and preferences [2, 4, 5, 6, 8]. Compared to other computer network like SeniorNet, ComputerLink has the following advantages: 1) participation does not require caregivers to leave home, 2) it can be accessed any time day or night, 3) use can be anonymous or self-identified and 4) information can be tailored to individual needs [2]. The ComputerLink project included several sub-projects, which addressed different research questions. Overall, these studies have demonstrated that "computers could become useful home care support mechanisms for patients and their caregivers to obtain information, peer support, and professional assistance and the innovative technologies would not be a problem even for people inexperienced with computers use." "ComputerLink represents an innovation that provides relative advantages over face-to-face social support interventions since the users can access the information and support at their own rate of interest, skill and style" [5, 6, 7]. Moreover, the ComputerLink was reported to be helpful in increasing confidence in patients' and caregivers' decision making [7], reducing caregivers' strain [2] and alleviating their emotional burden [11].

White and Dorman examined the content and themes of 532 messages posted on The Alzheimer Mailing List (www.adrc.wustl.edu/ALZHEIMER) during 20 days of 1998 and categorized all messages into eight subject areas: information giving/information seeking, encouragement/support, personal experience, personal opinion, prayer, thanks, humor and miscellaneous. Information giving and seeking were the major part of postings to the Alzheimer List followed by experiences and opinions sharing in number of postings. The members of the mailing list also tended to use the mailgroup to seek encouragement. According to White and Dorman, the Alzheimer List could bring several advantages compared to traditional support groups. For example, the mailing list provided opportunities for caregivers to vent feelings of grief, frustration, anger, and helplessness by writing, which would be especially useful for a private, reserved, shy person or during those moments when caregivers preferred not to make themselves the center of attention. Online support groups also provide members with an immediate opportunity to communicate their concerns with other members, so that they do not have to wait until the next meeting of a traditional support group or until a physician's office opens the next morning. White and Dorman suggested that "by becoming aware of the potential advantages that online support groups offer to caregivers, nurses can encourage Alzheimer caregivers to use online groups as an empowering and practical adjunct to traditional caregiver support" [23].

1. Problem Statement

The amount of research for Alzheimer's caregiving does not match the rapid growth of people with the disease or their caregivers. The PEW foundation has studied how Americans use the Internet in their daily life. However, caregivers of people with Alzheimer's disease are a unique group. Disruptive behaviors are common among individuals with Alzheimer's disease [20]. The caregiver's situation is compounded by an ongoing fear that the person with Alzheimer's disease will hurt herself/himself inadvertently. Thus caregivers are always on alert to protect the safety of their loved ones, and this continued alertness creates substantial mental tension and stress. The demanding nature of providing care changes the family caregivers' whole life which is different from other on-line populations. Understanding how caregivers of people with Alzheimer's disease use the Internet could suggest ways to maximize the potential of employing the Internet to improve their quality of life.

Brennan [7] and White and Dorman [23] studied an Alzheimer's website service, which mainly focused on providing health care/disease related information, disease treatment information and/or answers and solutions to some concerns emerging during the caregiving process. However, the Internet is multi-functioned. According to PEW Internet and American Life project, nearly all Internet users go online to conduct some of their ordinary day-to-day activities, from mundane tasks to social arrangements to personal recreation. The online activities can be divided into four categories: information seeking, communications, transactions and entertainment [18]. The Internet could affect caregiver's characteristics by changing their ways of conducting life tasks, including work, leisure and socialization, not just home care related activities. We need to understand the current use of the Internet in caregiver's daily life. This study is related to a larger project aimed at systematically exploring current use of the Internet among caregivers of persons with Alzheimer's disease, what factors affect the use of the Internet, caregivers' attitude toward the Internet and its impact on their life, and caregivers' perception of how the Internet could be used as a potential tool to assist them in home care. In this study, Internet use was examined both for access to disease-related information and services, and also for entertainment and communication with the outside world. This study sought to provide a complete and detailed view of the application of the Internet in different areas of caregivers' lives, including their work, leisure, socialization and emotional status, and personal care related tasks.

2. Previous research -- Caregivers' Online Activities

In previous research, an in-depth descriptive analysis was conducted with a small number of Internet users, who were also caregivers of persons with Alzheimer's disease. We identified the participants' online activities in five categories: Information Seeking, Communication, Online Transaction, Entertainment and Work-Related Activities. The last category overlapped with the first four. It turned out that the most popular online activities reported were online communication and information seeking. Eighty percent of the interviewees had looked for answers to specific questions about a broad variety of issues from health care to religion to news. The interviewees valued everyday communications on the Internet very high. Email was the dominant activity in this category and it was also one of the first activities that most interviewees tried as new users of the Internet. Participants did not often seek entertainment over the Internet, nor did they perform many work-related activities at home via the Internet.

During the interviews, the participants were specifically asked whether they used the Internet to assist their caregiving tasks. They used the Internet in the following ways: seeking medical or health care related information for Alzheimer's disease, seeking psychosocial support, contacting health professionals, facilitating coordination among family caregivers, releasing stress with online entertainment and entertaining the patient with online games, articles or mind teasers such as word puzzles.

3. Purpose and Method of Current Study

The aim of the current study was to explore how caregivers of persons with Alzheimer's disease obtain resources for their regular online activities, especially how they conduct online searches for desired information. The limited amount of research on use of the Internet among caregivers of persons with Alzheimer's disease, suggested the use of an exploratory approach. It was difficult to create detailed and structured hypotheses and questionnaires for a quantitative study based on the currently available literature. The data collected and analyzed in this study consisted primarily of the perspectives of Alzheimer's caregivers, communicating as positioned subjects, regarding their encounters and interactions with the Internet. In a positioned-subject approach, "subjects" refers to people with particular needs and "position" refers to the environment in which they are located [9]. The positioned subject approach focuses on people's positioned understandings and interpretations of their experiences and seeks to accurately characterize and synthesize positioned subjects' perspectives into a composite portrait.

We recruited our study participants through the Memory Research Program at the Madison Veterans Hospital and Alzheimer's Association South Central Wisconsin Chapter, located in Madison, Wisconsin. Ten participants were included in this study (mean age = 65 years, SD = 12 years), three male and seven female. Six of them were spouse caregivers (mean age = 72.2 years, SD = 8.9 years) and four were adult children caring for their parent (mean age = 54.3 years, SD = 6.7 years). Nine participants were caring for an individual with Alzheimer's disease when the interviews were conducted. Only one participant was a previous caregiver, whose mother was institutionalized in October 2003. Nine interviewees had been using the Internet for five years or longer. One subject started to use the Internet regularly about one year ago although he was introduced to it five years ago. All of the interviewees spent at least two hours online per week. Half of the participants self rated their computer skills as fair, three as proficient and two as poor.

Face-to-face interviews were conducted with a semi-structured interview script. Three pilot interviews were conducted to refine the interview questions. Before the interview, there was a 30-minute prescreening phone conversation, collecting the potential participants' demographic information and to determine their eligibility for this study. Follow-up phone calls were used to collect information missed during the interviews.

4. Results

There were four approaches for the interviewees to seek resources for their regular online activities: 1) resources provided by the interviewees' favorite website or the site they already knew; 2) resources from professional training; 3) resources provided by friends/family members; 4) keyword search of the desired topics. The participants also showed different behaviors to retrieve the useful resources after they found them: they could get the resources from their favorite websites; they bookmarked the resources; they memorized the addresses; or they memorized the keywords to get the resources through search engine again.

The interviewees usually started the information search with search engines like Yahoo or Google or with their preferred or recommended resources, which included their favorite websites or some resources they were aware of, for example, the websites recommended by those reputable websites they trusted, like America Online (AOL), Mayo Clinic, Heath Pro and the Alzheimer's Association. Preferred or recommended resources also included seeking information by emailing health professionals or other people who might have the answer, or posting questions on a message board and waiting for other board attendees to provide information.

The only two search engines used were Yahoo and Google. When the Google/Yahoo search did not lead to the desired answer, sometimes they turned to their preferred or recommended resources. When the search with the preferred or recommended resources did not provide satisfactory answers, they could refine the search keyword based on the related materials found through the preferred or recommended resources. The second option was not always available. The following example illustrates how the interviewees used the online keyword search:

> *I will search the Internet using keyword. I usually use Google or Yahoo. Most of the time it will bring up thousands of links and I have to narrow down from there...... But if I can't find the information I want by Google or Yahoo searching, I will go to some specific sites I knew or I saved before. I will start with the previous keyword – say "high blood pressure". Usually those sites are good with trustable information. At least they will provide me more keywords that I can use to search further, if not the information I need.*

Sometimes the participants initiated the information search by looking through the pre-filtered resources. If the preferred or recommended resources could not provided a satisfactory answer, Google/Yahoo keyword search was tried next.

Most interviewees used these two search approaches in combination. Their experience with the Internet and familiarity with the search topic seemed to be a factor affecting their choice of which path to take. When the search topic was something the interviewees had been through many times, it was likely that they already knew where to look for good information and they usually started with their favorite websites. However, when the search topic was something new or unfamiliar to them, they started with a search engine. When the participants were not skillful with a computer and the Internet, or they were not confident in their skill in finding desired information online, they would reduce their needs or limit the search to the resources with which they were familiar.

Often the online keyword search would bring up results. Some interviewees had their own approach to narrowing down the search results. The common strategies were judging the reputation of the website by its domain or reading the short description below the link.

5. Discussion and New Sights for Research

Some findings in this study are consistent with the literature. The two commonly used search engines reported were Yahoo and Google, similar to the PEW Foundation Internet study: "Internet users behave conservatively as searchers: they tend to settle quickly on a single search engine and then stick with it, rather than switching as search technology evolves or comparing results from different search systems. All of the participants regularly used just one or two engines. Yahoo and Google are the most popular search engine they used"[17].

Six participants used a keyword search to get the resources they needed. Web designers need to make their websites easily locatable by search engines selecting self-explanatory keywords. We would suggest website designers test their websites with Google and Yahoo before launching them to see if they could be found by keyword search, how many keywords could be used to locate them. Some participants believed that "the deeper you go down, the farther you are away from what you are asking for at the beginning".

The fact that some participants received information about the online resources from their friends or family is meaningful to website designers as well. This finding addresses the importance of a friendly technology environment.

The participants also received online resources from professional training and their favorite websites. This indicates the value of maintaining a good network with other agencies and organizations in the area to strengthen the outreach effort. It is helpful to increase the awareness and usage of the website or service by having visitors redirected through other sites.

References

[1] Balas, E., Austin, S., Mitchell, J., Ewigman, B., Bopp, K. and Brown, G. The clinical value of computerized information systems. *Archives of Family Medicine.* (1996). 5. 271–278.

[2] Bass, D., McClendon, M., Brennan, P. and McCarthy, C. The buffering effect of a computer support network on caregiver strain. Journal of Aging and Health. (1998). 10(1). 20-43.

[3] Beard, C., Kokmen, E., O'Brien, P. and Kurland, L. (1995). The prevalence of dementia is changing over time in Rochester, Minnesota. *Neurology*.1995. 45. 75-79.

[4] Brennan, P. and Moore, S. Networks for home care support: The ComputerLink project. *Caring.* (1994). 13. 64–70.

[5] Brennan, P., Moore, S. and Smyth, K. ComputerLink: Electronic support for the home caregiver. Advances in Nursing Science. (1991). 13(4). 14- 27

[6] Brennan P., Moore S. and Smyth K. Alzheimer's disease caregivers' uses of a computer network. *Western Journal of Nursing Research.* (1992). 14. 662–673.

[7] Brennan, P., Moore, S. and Smyth, K. The effects of a special computer network on caregivers of persons with Alzhermei's disease. Nursing Research. (1995). 44(3). 166-172

[8] Brennan, P. and Ripich, S. Use of a home-care computer network by persons with AIDS. International Journal of Technology Assessment in Health Care. (1994).10. 258-272.

[9] Conrad, C., Haworth, J. and Millar, S. (1993). *A silent success: master's education in the United States.* Baltimore: John Hopkins University Press.

[10] Evans, D., Scherr, P. and Cook, N. et al. Estimated prevalence of Alzheimer's disease in the United States. Milbank Q. (1990). 68. 267-289.

[11] Gallienne, R., Moore, S. and Brennan, P. Alzheimer's caregivers, psychosocial support via computer networks. Journal of Gerontological Nursing. (1993). 19(12).
[12] Haley, W. The family caregiver's role in Alzheimer's disease. Neurology. (1997). 48(5).
[13] Haley, W., West, C. and Wadley, V. et al. Psychological, social, and health impact of caregiving: a comparison of black and white dementia family caregivers and noncaregivers. Psychol Aging. (1995). 10. 540-552.
[14] Hebert, L., Scherr, P., Bienias, J., Bennett, D. and Evans, D. Alzheimer Disease in the U.S. Population: Prevalence Estimates Using the 2000 Census." Archives of Neurology August (2003). 60 (8). 1119 – 1122.
[15] Kiecolt-Glaser, J., Dura, J., Speicher, C., Trask, O. and Glaser, R. Spousal caregivers of dementia victims: longitudinal changes in immunity and health. Psychosom Med .(1991). 53. 345-362.
[16] Krishna, S., Balas, A., Spencer, D., Griffin, J. and Boren, S. Clinical trials of interactive computerized patient education: Implications for family practice. *The Journal of Family Practice.* (1997). 45. 25–33.
[17] PEW Internet and American Life Project. (2004). The Internet and Daily Life. http://www.pewinternet.org/pdfs/PIP_Internet_and_Daily_Life.pdf
[18] Schulz, R., Lusting, A., Handler, S. and Martire, L. Technology – based caregiver intervention research: current status and future directions. Gertontechnology. (2002). 2(1). 15-47.
[19] Semple, S. Conflict in Alzheimer's caregiving families: Its dimensions and consequences. The Gerontologist. (1992). 32. 656 – 664.
[20] Swearer, J. (1992). Behavioral disturbances in dementia. In: *Handbook of Dementing Illnesses.* New York, NY: Marcel Dekker; 1992.
[21] U.S. Congress, office of technology assessment. (1990). Confused minds, burdened families: finding helps for people with Alzheimer's and other dementia. (Report NO:OTA-BA-403). Washington, DC: US, Government Printing Office
[22] Venkatesh, V. and Davis, F. D. A theoretical extension of the Technology Acceptance Model: Four longitudinal field studies. Management Science. (2000). 46(2), 186-204.
[23] White, M. and Dorman, S. Online support for caregivers. Analysis of an Internet Alzheimer mailgroup. Computers in Nursing. (2000). 18(4). 168-76.
[24] Wright, L., Bennet, G., and Gramling, L. Telecommunication interventions for care-givers of elders with dementia. Advances in Nursing Science. (1998). 20(3). 76-88.

Promoting Independence for Older Persons with Disabilities
W.C. Mann and A. Helal (Eds.)
IOS Press, 2006

Technology Lab on a Shoestring: Developing Low Cost Evaluation Centers and Lending Libraries

Bob UTLEY[a]
[a]*Rehabilitation Technology Lab for Blindness and Low Vision, Oklahoma City, OK USA*

Abstract. Assistive Technology (AT) demonstration and evaluation centers are necessary for the accurate dissemination of information to the consumer and to verify the kinds of tools that would best suit the needs of the disabled. Evaluation and demonstration labs are often not available due to perceived costs. The need to "try before you buy" is also a very important aspect of proper AT provision. This paper describes the Oklahoma model showing low-cost ways of providing these services.

Keywords. Assistive technology, demonstration and evaluation centers

Introduction

In 1995 Oklahoma had five assistive technology specialists to serve our 77 counties, but we had no adaptive technology to demonstrate. We would schedule our AT evaluations in field offices to use our blind colleague's assistive devices. Our attempt was gallant, but woefully inadequate. Oklahoma Rehab seriously needed a technology demonstration and evaluation lab.

In April 1997 I accepted the challenge to grow a technology lab. There was only one catch—we had very little seed money, and almost no space. My office and lab would be housed in a single room at the Oklahoma Library for the Blind and Physically Handicapped. It was a 12' by 20', and when I moved in there was no furniture, no phone, and no door. I was given $25,000 to buy furniture, software, computers, electronic magnifiers, and any other tools I needed. We opened the evaluation lab on August 1, 1997 with the following tools: a laptop computer with a TFT 12" screen, a desktop computer with a 15" monitor, video magnifier with SVGA capabilities, one screen reading software, one screen enlargement software, and one talking note taking device.

Today, the Technology Lab for Blindness and Low Vision in the Oklahoma Library for the Blind and Physically Handicapped has about 20 various brands, sizes and types of electronic magnifiers that are supplied by 5 vendors. There is a 12-station training lab complete with various brands of optical character recognition software, screen readers and magnification programs. We also have several note-taking devices some with refreshable Braille, some without.

We wanted to add a training module to our program, but we needed more tools. We increased capital expenditures last year with additional funding of $50,000. As of

1997 our agency has invested $75,000 in the lab, but we display more than twice that amount in technology value. The question, then, is "how do we display $150,000 worth of product on a $75,000 investment?"

1. Help Was Offered

Tulsa is home to three of the best technology vendors in the country. There is steep competition among them. One vendor wanted his electronic magnifier on display in the lab, and offered to loan us one. My administration approved the vendor's offer, but cautioned me that no promotion of one machine over another would be allowed.

Within weeks, all of our vendors provided us with "loaner" tools. I wrote to companies that produce adaptive technology for the blind. I explained what we were trying to do and explained we needed their help. I told them we were willing to take older versions of software or demo copies. We had a very positive response.

We had companies send us full-blown versions of adaptive software, and one company sent a complete computer system with adaptive software loaded and ready to use. The national vendors met my request with unbelievable acceptance. Everyone understood that we would not "sell" their equipment for them. All we would do is demonstrate it and let consumers "try on the tools for size."

2. Beg, Borrow, and Steal!

Here are some things we have done others could replicate. First check that your state laws will permit some of the things we have done.

1. Invite Vendors to Place Tools in the Lab. Caution the vendors that they cannot expect you to "push" their product. Some vendors have removed tools because they did not feel we were "supporting their products" as much as we should. Vendors who expect us to help sell their products are invited to remove their tools from the lab.
2. Accept Donations of Used Equipment. Some states have laws against state agencies receiving donations, but most state agencies have community support organizations that can accept contributions. Donations to the technology lab have been made to the "Friends of the Library" who then can place them in our care.
3. Dead Client Surplus. The name is dreadful, but it is fact. Clients die, and often the adaptive tools come back to the agency. The money used to purchase adaptive tools for clients was client services money. Therefore it must remain in client services. When our lab was new, we used these tools as much as we could. However, when another consumer needed them, we had to give them up. Now, we often keep these tools separate and apart from the lab tools and we use them primarily for loan.
4. Warehouse Scavenger. Agency administration said no adaptive technology would be sent to surplus auctions. All of our retired technology was sent to our warehouse. Recently I transferred several retired magnifiers, computers, software and other adaptive tools from the warehouse to the technology lab. Much of it is junk, but there were a few older style video magnifiers in the

mix that we can loan if we are in a bind. We also discovered that we could mix and match parts from various machines to get one usable tool from a pile of parts. In one instance the consumer had an old Windows 95 computer. We had an old copy of a screen reading program that worked perfectly with her old computer. We recycled that tool back to the consumer.

5. Grants. At the end of this document is a recounting of how we received a grant to buy assistive technology for our program, and the funds to develop an entirely new program for lending.
6. Tech Act Office. Every state has a tech act office. Approach them for tools to demonstrate in your lab. They may be loaners and they may be there for short periods of time, but you may be able to use them for a while.
7. Use Field Offices. As we did in the beginning, find offices around your state that have adaptive technology in use. Ask your colleagues if they will let you use their tools so you can do an evaluation. We have even called former clients and asked them if we could use their technology to demonstrate the technology to a person who lives in their town. Most are more than willing to help, and they love the attention.
8. Tools from Retired Colleagues. When a colleague retires or resigns, they may be leaving behind some hardware and software that you could use in your lab. I lay claim to any and all technology not in use in our agency.
9. Approach Business Leaders. We approached our lead employer with the Business Leadership Network and told him we wanted to network the computers in our training room. He not only gave us the router, but he paid for our DSL drop.

3. Demonstration or Training:

In March 2003, we opened our training center at the Technology Lab. As we discussed the addition of a training module to our program, we began to understand the difference between a demonstration lab and a training center.

Part of our capital upgrades last year included 3 desktop computers and 4 laptops, but we needed more. We approached our agency's IT department and asked for any computers they were not using. They gave us six desktop computers from 3 to 5 years old. We now have a mixture of Windows 98, 2000, NT and XP in the training room, but each machine has up-to-date screen reading, magnification and OCR programs

Training centers require current adaptive tools. We may be using some systems that are out dated, (for example, Windows 98), but adaptive technology must be as current as possible. Our consumers may use Windows 98 on the job, and many consumers have older systems in their homes. Therefore, it does not disturb us to have a few older computer systems in our training lab, because this is what our consumers have.

Evaluation programs do not need the most current versions of adaptive software. The primary event in demonstrations and evaluations is determining what the consumer can see, or what they can hear. Older versions of technology will help the consumer understand the concept of the technology being recommended, and can be used to evaluate the consumer's ability to use those tools.

If you need demonstration and evaluation tools, start talking about your need to your administration, colleagues, former clients, friends, vendors, manufacturers and business leaders. Don't be afraid to dig in the warehouse for out dated tools. They don't have to be brand new to answer the big questions.... How well can the consumer see the screen? AND/OR... How well can the consumer hear the speech?

4. Lending Library Development

In the fall of 2003 the Visual Services Division of the State of Oklahoma's Department of Rehabilitation Services embarked on a grant writing project to help move the agency toward a lending library for the blind and visually impaired consumers of the agency.

We started the grant writing with the ultimate end of a $150,000 project that would serve the Oklahoma City area. The process proved beneficial, but time consuming. We were not experienced in writing grants. So, much of our time for the first year was spent in learning how to proceed with the technical aspects of such a project. Our agency administrator contracted with the grant writer from a local University to help us understand the process and to teach us how to write our proposal.

In the spring of 2004 we were very near the end of our grant writing and knew we would be looking for potential grantors in the coming few weeks. We began our research to find a grantor(s) who we would approach for the assistance. We knew our own agency would help with some investment money to prove our intentions worthy, but we really needed a substantial investment from someone that would believe in us enough to help us start this worthy project.

In the fall of 2004 we learned that the Tech Act office in Oklahoma (Oklahoma AbleTech, Stillwater, OK) was interested in talking to us. They had been instructed that part of their funds were to fund "try before you buy" programs. We began our negotiations with AbleTech in January of 2005.

The Visual Services division agreed to focus on this program as a positive investment in our citizens with disabilities. The funds available were nearly $80K. This included $12,500 for the Oklahoma School for the Blind and the Oklahoma School for the Deaf to fund Lending Libraries and try-before-you-buy-programs as well. As both of the schools are part of the Vocational Rehabilitation agency, we all worked collaboratively to see this project to the end.

One of the primary hurdles we had to overcome was the fact that the Vocational Rehabilitation programs in the state of Oklahoma are designed as an "employment agency" for individuals with disabilities. The Oklahoma AbleTech had intentions for us to serve anyone from the "cradle to the grave". We had to connect with the staff to come up with plans to accommodate this change in our scope of services. The local Vocational Rehab agency does have transition programs, and both of the schools under our umbrella, so we did have some outlets to provide services to those below and above the working age of our consumers. We also had, at the time of the grant preparation, an older blind program that served individuals who, without our help, were at risk for institutionalization. The plan started to come together.

We began to recognize that we would need additional staff to help with the lending program. A "SWIP" worker (State Worker Incentive Program) was hired to help develop this program.

On August 17, 2005 we took a moving truck to Stillwater and picked up our lending library tools. At the writing of this document, we are unpacking, bar-coding, organizing, and loading the adaptive software for these tools to be loaned.

5. Specifics for our Lending Library Program:

For eight years we were a technology lab for blindness and low vision products. We provided onsite, home, and worksite evaluations and demonstrations. We did loan tools, but those came from client surplus supply and various other places. We were not set up to meet the needs of everyone who walked through our doors.

We knew Assistive Technology for Blindness and Low Vision. We thought it better to limit the kinds of tools we had and prove total competencies rather than have an across the board smattering of all kinds of technology for all kinds of disabilities and run the risk of not being able to serve anyone with any level of proficiency. It was decided that the technology lending lab would have tools we knew best. Therefore, the lending library only has technology for blindness and low vision related issues. Oklahoma AbleTech has told us that we can re-apply for more funds next year and we can then discuss branching out into other disability related areas.

Since adaptive/assistive technology for those who are blind (especially) and low vision often have a solid learning curve attached to them, it was decided before anyone left our office with loaned tools, they would be trained on the use of those tools.

Two examples:

1. If we loan an electronic magnifier (closed circuit TV reading machine) we will sit with the consumer and make sure they totally understand how it functions and how to adjust it for their specific needs. Once they prove able to adequately use the machine, then it will be sent with them or delivered by our staff as soon as possible.
2. If we loan a computer with talking software, we assess the consumer's computer skills and abilities, keyboarding skills, and then determine what kind of talking software will most appropriately meet their needs.

Sending a consumer home with a piece of equipment that they cannot use can be as detrimental as the initial loss of their vision, or even possibly more detrimental. Without proper training, the hope they had in the technology soon dissipates and they again feel they are at the "dead-end" to rehabilitative recovery. Therefore, no adaptive tool and or software will leave this library without a clear concept of what they will be able to accomplish with the tool, and proof they either know how to use it, or there is in place a training plan to teach them how to use it.

6. Conclusion

Oklahoma has invested time, effort, money, energy and manpower into the development of one of the finest assistive technology programs (via a state rehab agency) in the country. We feel we have the consumers of the agency at center of our program, we have the scope and services of the agency guiding our actions and we have the faith and investment of the state Tech Act office standing close in partnership with us in our program.

Promoting Independence for Older Persons with Disabilities
W.C. Mann and A. Helal (Eds.)
IOS Press, 2006

In Brief:

Using Videophones as an Antidote to Isolation of the Elderly and a Learning Tool for the Young

Saul B. Troen, Ph.D.

Introduction

The purpose of this paper is to describe the results of a "Living and Learning Legacy" intergenerational program that introduced videophone virtual visitations to enhance the quality of life of the aged in a long term care residential facility and, at the same time, provide middle school children with an appreciation of their life and meaning.

Videophone technology played an integral role in this program because society and culture has traditionally been based on face-to-face communication. The "Living and Learning Legacy" program is important because the addition of a visual component to an ordinary telephone conversation increased the bonding between the "grandparent" and "grandchild".

1. Background

Feelings of loneliness and isolation often due to the lack of social contact frequently occur in older persons. Studies indicate that social interaction, even at a minimum, is critical for helping to maintain and improve a person's well being [1]. While writing letters enables communication, it is limited in time and space; letters do not provide visual or auditory contact. While television fills the role of immediacy, it does not provide for reciprocal communication. The telephone, on the other hand, provides for instant auditory communication. While the sound of a voice can be comforting, it has its limitations. It does not provide a visual stimulus and face-to-face communication.

Numerous studies have been done that measure the independent and interactive relationships of social support networking on mental and physical health of the elderly. Studies using videoconferencing usually focus on the use of videoconferencing as a solution for augmenting the health of patients living in their own homes or for the exchange of information between different sites.

While it is known that loneliness and isolation can contribute to the need for more intensive care it appears that little attention has been given on using videoconferencing to eliminate loneliness and isolation.

The goal of the "Living and Learning Legacy Program" based on the "Adopt a Grandparent" is two fold. Through technological skills learned throughout the year, the students developed a bond with the residents at the Atria Senior Living Community Center in Kew Gardens, NY. The students learned interview skills, how to write reports and newsletters on the information they obtained. The girls were able to communicate with residents without leaving the classroom. They learned how to use technology and multimedia to interpret and record information.

The residents at the Atria had an opportunity to pass along their ideologies and experiences to the students. The "Living and Learning Legacy" played an important role in providing the participants with a useful activity that generated greater self worth and esteem. It also alleviated feelings of isolation.

After two years of operation, the program had succeeded beyond expectations. The "Living and Learning Legacy" not only enhanced the quality of life of the elderly participants but the students involved in the project learned from the older participants in ways not anticipated. We did not anticipate the depth of the feelings the students would have from their encounter with the elderly.

2. The Participants

The ordinary adopt-a-grandparent program establishes a special one-to-one relationship between an elderly person living either at home or in a local nursing care facility and a volunteer. Although the needs of the seniors may vary, each volunteer is meant to be a much-needed friend and companion to his or her "grandparent".

This particular "Living and Learning Legacy" program differs from the Adopt-A-Grandparent program in that it is a school wide project and incorporates video technology.

The school, the Bnos Malka Academy of Queens, New York, is an all girls private school. The Atria of Kew Gardens was chosen as the long term care facility because the vice principle would often visit the residents.

The administration of the school incorporated this project into its "Hesed" or "good deeds" curriculum. This program fit the school's philosophy of having the students do "good deeds" and at the same time provides them with an understanding of how changing technologies may impact their future.

The 6th, 7th, and 8th grade girls participated in the program. Before beginning the program, the students were prepared in class what it means to be an 'adopted grandchild'. After this introduction, they were introduced to the videophone and its operation. The students became very excited with the prospect of using video-telephones on a regular basis to supplement personal visits. The 8th grade girls also decided that their graduation project would be to present to their parents what they learned and felt being an "adopted grandchild".

3. Summary

The use of videophones as an antidote to isolation of older adults and as a learning tool for the young warrants more study. Videophones can serve as an important bridge between generations. The impact of videoconferencing on intergenerational interaction is not well documented and doing so may provide expanded ways of enhancing the well-being and quality of life of the elderly and, at the same time, enable children to appreciate older adults.

References

[1] Tsirakis, T (1999), Social interaction improves mental and physical well being. Originally published in: Geriatrics and Aging, 2, (5). September/October www.geriatricsandaging.ca. Retrieved November 5, 2002 from the World Wide Web.

Chapter 3

Housing, Home Modifications and Universal Design

Promoting Independence for Older Persons with Disabilities
W.C. Mann and A. Helal (Eds.)
IOS Press, 2006

Design and Construction of a Universal Cabinet Prototype

David RINGHOLZ [a,1]
[a]*Georgia Institute of Technology, Industrial Design, Atlanta, GA*

Abstract. This paper documents the design and production of a Universal Cabinet concept created for use in the kitchen and bath. In order to address the needs of a broad range of stakeholders, including users, builders, developers and manufacturers, this functional prototype integrates a height adjustable work surface, clear knee space and requires no specialized modification for installation. To facilitate technology transfer, it has been refined and constructed using the latest Computer Numeric Controlled machine technology.

Keywords. Universal design, cabinet design, clear knee space

1. Background

The intent of the Universal Cabinet Project is to develop kitchen and lavatory cabinetry suitable for general use that also meets State and Federal Accessibility requirements without specialized installation or modification. A1989 amendment to Title VIII of the Civil Rights Act of 1968 "The Fair Housing" Act, contains design and construction accessibility provisions for certain new multifamily dwellings developed for first occupancy on or after March 13, 1991. Most developers respond to accessibility requirements by specifying "accessible" products for installation into some portion of the environment. For example, a multi-family housing developer must designate a certain percentage of the dwelling units as accessible. For these units he is forced to select from a small supply of commercially available products that meet accessibility requirements and are not suitable for installation into the remaining dwellings. A universal cabinet that is functionally and aesthetically appropriate for all dwelling units, regardless of accessibility designation, would be a tremendous cost and time savings to the developer as well as a dramatic improvement on the overall performance of the environment.

North Carolina State University's Center for Universal Design generated early concepts to address this opportunity, in response to inquiries from a local developer. The need for this cabinet to accommodate seated and standing users necessitates flexibility in function which includes a height adjustable work surface and clear floor space beneath.

In order to be readily adopted by the housing industry, this cabinet must be priced competitively and require no additional labor to install. It was quickly determined that the integration of motorized parts or custom mechanisms would increase costs to prohibitive levels. Ideally this cabinet should be cost-competitive with mid-range commercial products.

The initial concept featured triangular wedge that moved up and down a given angle and achieved different vertical heights for the user. The concept was never modeled so the details of the proposed mechanism were not solved. The mechanism was a 'gear' that ran along a track with 'teeth.' A separate part with 'teeth' locked with the track at various points. The user lifted the front edge of the wedge and moved it up and down the track stopping at any point desirable. Since the 'teeth' were continuous there were no pre-determined heights.

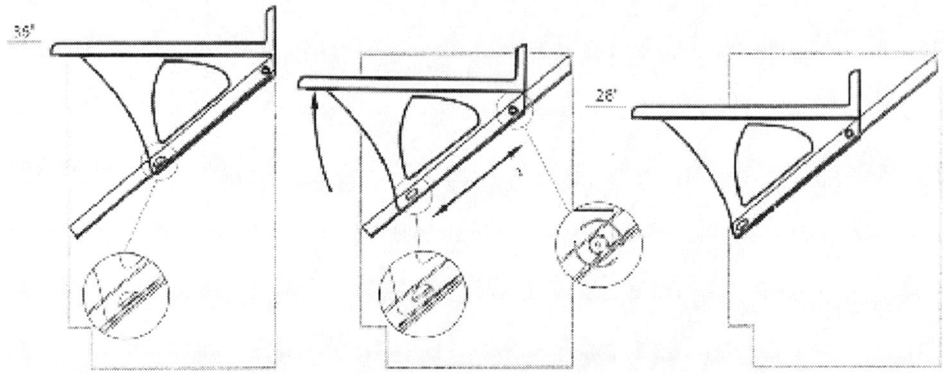

Figure 1. Adjustable height countertop mechanics

The follow-up concept developed by the Center for Universal Design also implemented the wedge concept. The cabinet had a very sturdy base to which the pocketing doors were mounted. The mechanism was a custom piece of hardware mounted on the outside of the cabinet base. An effective feature of this design was the permanent horizontal surface at 36." Although the cabinet worked as intended it was not practical for manufacturing purposes. The cabinet was an effective stand-alone custom solution but not realistic for integration in a kitchen environment. The cabinet can not be attached through traditional means to adjacent cabinets without large gaps between to allow for the mechanism.

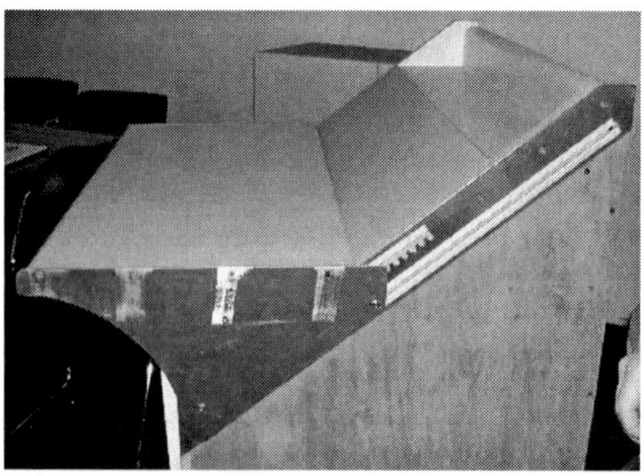

Figure 2. Prototype cabinet.

At this stage the cabinet could not have been readily adapted to standard commercial construction techniques. Therefore, the primary goal of the project from this point is to take this concept and refine it for mass production.

2. Criteria Development

Design criteria from the initial project were adapted and validated for guidance during this phase. Users, developers, builders and technicians contributed to the following design criteria. An effective product must:

- meet State and Federal Accessibility requirements without modification
- have a height adjustment from 30"-42."
- have a convertible floor for a user in a seated position.
- be manufactured in a CNC environment
- be price competitive with mid-range cabinet products
- Align with standard product aesthetic in this category
- be compatible with standard cabinet doors.
- require no special installation, no special training and no special tools.
- have no removable parts.
- be standard base kitchen cabinet dimensions.
- be adjustable manually; no motorized components.

3. Methods

In all six different prototypes were constructed, tested and refined to yield the final result. Early models were individually crafted to test mechanics, proportion, weight distribution and ease of use. These were subsequently refined to interface with the AWPL production infrastructure. The project ultimately yielded three fully functional prototypes.

3.1. Computer Numeric Control [CNC] Overview

A CNC router was identified as the most appropriate option for prototype construction. This machine facilitates the rapid and precise production necessary for cabinetry components. The CNC router utilizes a vacuum system that holds the material in place while cutting. The working table is stainless steel and the vacuum 'holes' are spaced three inches apart in both directions covering the four foot by eight foot table. The holes open to allow air through or close to prohibit does airflow depending upon the size the material. Medium Density Fiberboard (MDF) is an ideal material to use with this system because of its very porous nature. The air actually penetrates the board to create a great amount of suction. In simple terms, the CNC router cuts out shapes. The g-code programs are generated from AutoCAD (or other compatible application) files. The AutoCAD files are two dimensional profiles. Once the router is fed the g-code programs it cuts out the shapes as designed.

3.2. Prototype - Phase One

The first models produced were an exploration into the wedge; how it would travel and how it would stop at various heights. They were basic compared to the level of complexity they would ultimately reach. This phase focused on making the wedge lighter. The weight of the MDF necessitated significant material removal. Determining the wedge angle was a complicated activity that required simultaneous consideration of the amount of counter space, the distance of horizontal drift into kitchen space, level of manufacturing complexity and the weight of the moving part.

3.3. Prototype - Phase Two

The next iteration of modeling focused almost exclusively on the convertible floor which had very simple requirements. That is, the assumption is that the floor would be 'converted' less than five times during the cabinet's lifetime; therefore, a simple, lowest cost, least labor intensive solution is likely the best solution. It is necessary for the floor to collapse to provide clear knee space for a person in a seated position to use the counter surface.

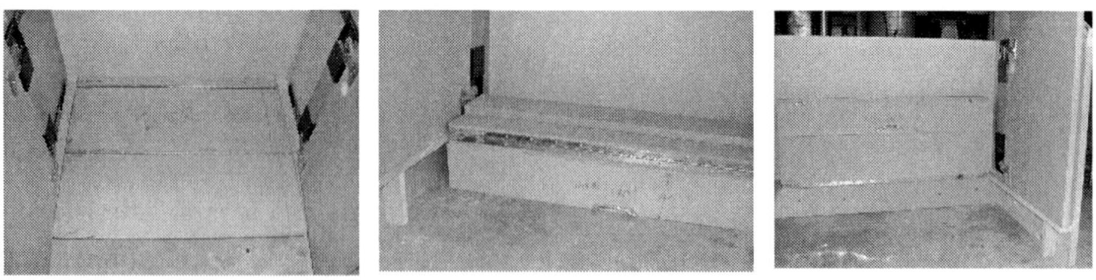

Figure 3. Early floor models

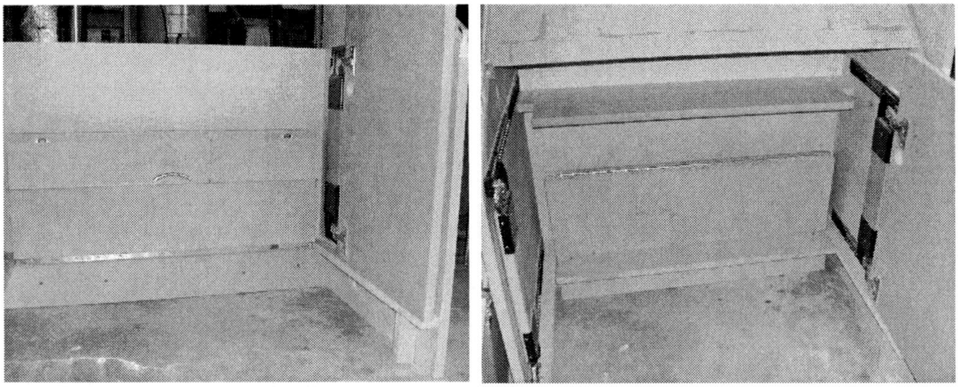

Figure 4. Next Generation Floor Models

The second approach was based on an accordion concept. In this solution the floor "breaks" in the middle forming an upside down "V". The challenge was getting the floor to "break" by pushing back on the top of the toe kick. An additional mechanism was required to achieve this.

The final floor solution was quite simple. The floor is lifted from the front edge and pushed up to the back wall. A task easily accomplished by hand, foot or through the use an assistive device. A piece of hardware attached to the front of the floor latches into its mate, which is mounted on the back wall.

3.4. Prototype - Phase Three

MDF proved to be an impractical solution for the wedge support rails since it is not durable enough to withstand the necessary friction. Hardwood was considered and modeled, though this solution requires lubrication. Also, wood is susceptible to expansion and contraction with changes in the weather. TIVAR® (Tough Inert Very Abrasion Resistant) was chosen for the final prototype. It is a brand name for UHMW-PE (Ultra High Molecular Weight Polyethylene), or UHMW. Its key properties are high abrasion resistance, natural lubrication, high impact strength, chemical resistance, corrosion resistance, moisture resistance and acoustic impedance. Additionally, UHMW is very easy to machine. TIVAR® is an expensive material ($250.00 for a 2' x 4' sheet 1.75 inch thick) but its properties are very attractive for this application. Compared to other UHMW materials such as Noryl, Ultem® and Delrin® TIVAR® is the least expensive.1 In fact, in most cases it will outlast Nylon, Teflon® and Acetal. The properties that make TIVAR appropriate for this application present other challenges. No glue, wood glue or epoxy will adhere to it. 5mm dowel holes were ultimately utilized and necessary for exact alignment of the rails. Once in place, counter bores were drilled to use screws as the new method of attachment.

4. Results

As with any design project, the outcomes can be evaluated by the degree to which they meet the established design criteria. In most cases the Universal Cabinet meets or exceeds the specifications set forth by the design criteria.

The final prototype is constructed of Medium Density Fiberboard [MDF], laminated with white Melamine. It measures 33inches in width, which is one typical measurement for standard kitchen base cabinets. This is the minimum width that will meet the Federal Accessibility requirement of 30 inch clear knee space for seated users.

Though the cabinet can be manufactured at any width, the knee space would be compromised at measurements below 33 inches.

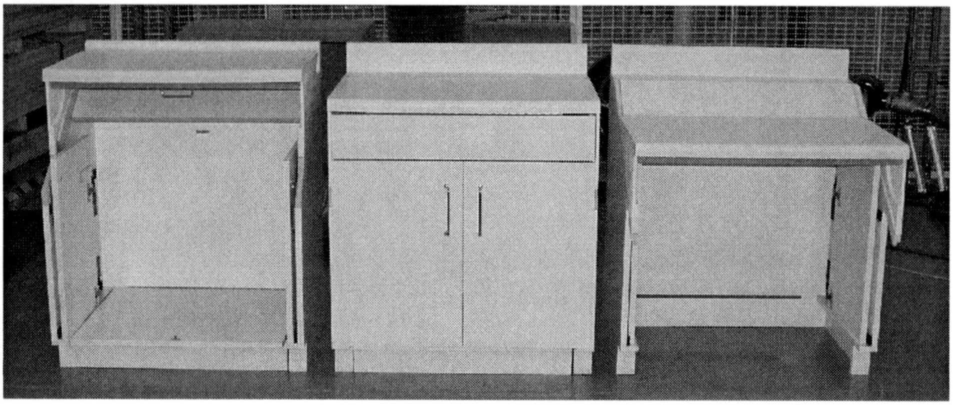

Figure 5. Final cabinet prototype.

Due to mechanical restrictions, the work surface height does not meet the initially specified metric, but it does adjust, manually from 30 inches to 39 inches. This is still a significant accomplishment and well below the 44 inch accessibility requirement, for seated users. The 3 inch adjustment above the standard counter height of 36 inches is very comfortable for tall, standing users.

The floor folds easily to accommodate seated users. The latch mechanism holds the floor securely to the rear wall of the cabinet, eliminating the need to make it removable.

The cabinet parts are arranged on a 48 inch by 96 inch piece of MDF using a computer application to optimize positioning for maximum efficiency and minimum waste. The MDF is secured to a Computer Numeric Controlled Router by vacuum pressure before the machine traces tools paths specified by the CAD file.

5. Conclusions

This product has achieved the level of refinement required to satisfy functional and mass production integration requirements. This research program has contributed significantly to the evolution of the Universal Cabinet concept by supporting prototype development, construction and testing and critical transition between concept and production most often deemphasized in the academic environment. The prototypes generated by this project are intended to support linkages between academic research and regional commercial resources. It is likely that further design refinements will be suggested as the product is evaluated by users and cabinet makers for the purposes of ease of use and commercialization.

Promoting Independence for Older Persons with Disabilities
W.C. Mann and A. Helal (Eds.)
IOS Press, 2006

Home Modifications Down Under

Desleigh DE JONGE[a,1], Elizabeth AINSWORTH[a], Bronwyn TANNER[a]
[a]*Department of Occupational Therapy, University of Queensland, Brisbane, Australia*

Abstract. This paper will describe the policies which facilitate the provision of home modification services to older Australians. It will review the national and state based funding schemes which provide cost-free and low-cost home modification services and examine the nature and availability of these services. Research in Australia examining the nature of home modifications, design features associated with injuries and the efficacy of home modifications will also be discussed.

Keywords. Home modifications, universal design, legislation

Introduction

The role of the environment as a major factor in enabling or disabling the achievement of both daily activities and community participation has been well established. There is an increasing recognition in both the disability and aged care sectors of the importance of creating environments that facilitate equality of opportunity for active participation in social, cultural, economic and political aspects of society [34]. The home environment is central to the facilitation of effective participation and the modification of the home environment is increasingly recognized as an appropriate policy and practice response. Home modifications have been defined as conversions or adaptations to the permanent physical features of the home environment in order to reduce the demands from the physical environment and as a result, make tasks easier, reduce accidents and support independent living [18, 26]. There is an increasing recognition of the growth in the need and benefits of home modifications [17].

Home modification service provision in Australia is strongly influenced by national and state based legislation, policies and government funding programs. Australia has a health and welfare system that promotes equity and is designed to enable people to participate in the social and economic aspects of community life. It aims to provide people throughout Australia with equal access to affordable services and has developed specific services to address the needs of vulnerable people in the community such as the young people with disabilities, older people and indigenous Australians. It is a complex system, comprising many types of services with a range of funding and regulatory mechanisms [6]. A concern of the system however is that there is a lack of integration of such areas as housing, health, disability and aged care at a policy and practice level.

This paper describes population trends, legislative and policy responses and services supporting people in the home in Australia. In addition it will provide an overview of the outcomes of home modifications services.

1. Population Growth and Changes

Australia's population continues to grow. In various States around Australia, most populations congregate around the major cities. There have been population shifts towards the coastal strips, growth in inner city living and an expansion of outer suburbs within major cities. The majority of health services are located in the more densely populated areas of Australia. A significant and unprecedented population trend is the increasing ageing of Australia's population. The Australian population is ageing numerically, in that the number of older people is increasing and structurally, in that the proportion of people who are aged 65 years and older is rising. This has wide ranging implications for Australian society, particularly in the areas of employment, infrastructure, health and aged care services [7,8].

2. Disability, Ageing and Living Arrangements

According to the Australian Bureau of Statistics (ABS) Disability, Ageing and Carers Survey (DACS) [3], one in five people in Australia (3,958,300 or 20.0%) have a reported disability, with little variation in gender (males (19.8%) and females (20.1%). For those with a reported disability, where disability is defined as any limitation, restriction or impairment, which has lasted, or is likely to last, for at least six months and restricts everyday activities, 86% (3,387,900) were limited in the core activities of self care, mobility or communication. The rate of disability increases with age, reaching 92% for those aged 90 years and over [3].

Physical conditions were the most commonly reported main health conditions of persons with a disability (84%). The remaining 16% of the group are reported to have had a mental or behavioral disorder as their main condition [3].

The ABS DACS conducted in 1998 show that the majority of Australians (89%) live in a private home with at least one other person. This is also the case for three-quarters of people with disabilities. However, people with disabilities are more likely than others to live alone with nearly 18% of all people with disabilities residing by themselves, compared to 6% of those without a disability [3].For those with severe or profound restrictions, as many as one in eight people live alone and must rely on the support of carers coming into their home to remaining living independently [3]. The impact of living arrangements are greater for those in the 15 to 64 year age bracket, as for this group, 15% of those with severe or profound restrictions live alone compared to only 7% of those without a disability in the same age group [3]. This discrepancy is not present in people 65 years and older, as 20% of those with severe or profound restrictions live alone compared to 28% of those without a disability. Many older people living alone have a history of living in a family home, from which children have moved on and spouses or partners have died or needed out-of-home care.

As the incidence of disability is greater in the older age ranges, the trend of population ageing may have implications for the rate of disability in the Australian population. Overall in Australia in 2002, older people (65 years and over) comprised 13% of Australia's total population and this is projected to rise to 30% by 2051 [4]. According to the ABS [2] and the Australian Institute of Health and Welfare [7], the older person in Australia, is likely to:

- Live in a house, flat, unit or apartment (93.3%), with most (71.1%) living in a separate house;
- Have a variety of living arrangements with most living with a partner (59%) or other relatives (10%). Of the 21.7% of those who live alone, the majority women. This gender disparity increases with age;
- Be 'asset rich but income poor' with 75.5 % owning their own home outright, another 4.4% still making mortgage payments and 78% receiving a government allowance or pension as their primary source of income. Of those in private accommodation, only 5.2 % rent privately with 5.5% in public housing; and
- Have been born in Australia, however 30.5% of people over 65years will have been born overseas, many from culturally and linguistically diverse backgrounds. Of Indigenous Australians, only 2.8% are 65 years or older compared to nearly 13% of all Australians.

Population ageing is a major focus of social and economic planners and policy makers in Australia, with particular concern relating to the anticipated increase in costs associated with the care and income support of a rapidly growing aged population. Recent government policy initiatives have focused on cost reduction as well as shifting costs and responsibility from the public sector to individuals, families, community groups and private businesses [7].

3. Housing Trends in Australia

Australia has one of the highest rates of home ownership in the world with owner occupation being the main form of tenure (80%) [33].The demand for housing in Australia continues to grow however, due to factors such as cost, availability or adequacy, not all Australians will be able to secure housing in the private market.

Strong links between housing and health have also been well established with factors such as dwelling condition and tenure type impacting on health [7]. For older people in Australia, the group most at risk of not achieving successful ageing-in-place is older people who have a low income and who are dependent on public programs to provide the necessary assistance [21]. This has particular meaning when considering the majority of older Australians who are described as being 'asset rich but income poor' and who are currently living in homes on reasonably large blocks, that were first occupied decades earlier in post war suburbs. These were designed for families with private cars. Only small percentages are living in rental accommodation, with those in public housing rental (5.5%) only slightly higher than those in private rental (5.2%) [2, 19]. Many houses are also ageing, resulting in older people living in homes in various stages of dilapidation or with serious physical defects. Even for housing in good repair, the majority of private housing has design features such as stairs which, as their occupants' age, become safety hazards and barriers to independence [11].

4. Legislative and Policy Responses to Address Community Participation

In Australia, as in many other countries, policy concerning people with disabilities is expressed in terms of integration, full participation and equality. The basic philosophy of the Australian welfare system relates to providing a system of general support for society and supplementing it with support for individuals with disabilities. Australia has various pieces of legislation that have reinforced the need for people with disabilities to have the same opportunities and the same obligations as others in society. An outcome of the implementation of the various pieces of legislation has been the increasing emphasis on community care policy and service delivery of which home modification services are a part. A characteristic of much of the legislation is that it involves both Commonwealth and State levels of government in implementation of funding and service delivery.

4.1. Legislation in Relation to Disability

The Commonwealth Disability Services Act (1986), Commonwealth State/Territory Disability Agreement (2003), and the Disability Discrimination Act (1992), have all had significant impact on the policy direction of society as the rights of individuals with disabilities to live in the community have been acknowledged. The Commonwealth Disability Services Act (1986) and the Commonwealth State/Territory Disability Agreement (CSTDA) (2002-2007), provide a national policy framework for the Australian and State governments to fund, monitor and support quality services for people with a disability. Accommodation for younger people with disabilities is a State and Territory responsibility under the CSTDA.

The CSTDA reaffirms that the role of the various levels of government is to develop and deliver public policy and services and to promote the rights, equality of opportunity, citizenship and dignity of people with disabilities. Funding has been used in the last decade to move people from institutions into the community and to provide care through the supported accommodation program for people with various disabilities. These deinstitutionalisation policies resulted in significant government funding being dedicated to building and modifying homes to facilitate transition from congregated care to independent living. In some States, a small amount of funding has been made available for home modifications.

The Disability Discrimination Act (1992) is one of the major national expressions of the human rights approach to disability, making discrimination on the grounds of disability unlawful. The Act covers the needs of carers and is considered significant because it defines disability in the broadest sense to include any type of physical, emotional and/or intellectual impairment. The Act also classifies actions based on perceptions of impairment as discriminatory and makes it against the law to discriminate against someone if they have a disability in the areas of employment, education, access to premises, provision of goods, services and facilities, activities of clubs and associations, sport and accommodation. Developments in public access design have contributed to home modification design in domestic settings in the community. In addition, equitable access to accommodation underpins Commonwealth housing legislation.

4.2. Legislation in Relation to Housing and Home Modifications

The majority of housing assistance is provided for under the Commonwealth Housing Assistance Act (1996) and through the Commonwealth State Housing Agreement (CSHA) (2003 – 2008) which aims to guide the various State Housing Authorities around Australia on the use of funds to address the housing need of people whose needs cannot be adequately met in the private housing system; to ensure the provision of housing is not an end in itself but will produce other positive social outcomes and; to ensure that housing strategies are coordinated with other government policies to support individuals and communities.

Under the CSHA, funding assistance is provided through State-owned public housing which has been a key service in providing appropriate housing for people with disabilities on low incomes who are not homeowners through the provision of housing assistance for rental housing, home purchase and specific housing programs. While only housing a small percentage of the total number of people with disabilities and people 65years and over, public housing provides security of tenure not available in the private rental market. In recent times public housing has focused on a target population of people whose needs cannot be met adequately in the private rental market. Older persons with a disability account for 30% of public housing occupancies [11]. The total number of consumers with disabilities is not known due to a failure of some people to identify that they have a disability. The State Housing Authorities around Australia have established home modification and new construction programs to cater for the needs of those in state owned housing and some have taken the initiative to create products to suit the needs of this group living in private housing.

4.3. Legislation in Relation to Aged Care

In the mid 1980's the Australian Federal Government initiated a process of aged care reforms in response to the projected increase in the size of the older population and in recognition that older people prefer to remain living in their own homes. These reforms included the expansion of home-based care services and low-care/ hostel accommodation and a reduction in the proportion of older people being placed in nursing home accommodation [1]. The reforms attempted to provide improved coordination between housing and the aged care sectors in the hope of alleviating poor health, social isolation and premature entry to residential care [19]. Reforms to the aged care sector continued when in 1997, the Commonwealth Government of Australia introduced the Aged Care Act (1997) which heralded a package of reforms to the existing aged care industry including improvements in access to care for people who wish to be cared for in their own homes, through the increased provision of community care [20]. Since this time, the Commonwealth Government has developed the National Strategy for an Ageing Australia [8] that offers a framework for responding to the changes that the population ageing would bring [7]. The strategy concluded that the implications of the population ageing affects more than aged care service planning and provision and that a whole of government approach is required that considers policy issues and addresses the issues ageing raises for individuals and for the larger community [7].

There has been an increased emphasis on community care and a decreased emphasis on institutional care. This trend began with the creation of the Home and Community Care Act (1985) and the Commonwealth State/Territory Home and

Community Care Agreement. The Home and Community Care (HACC) Program is a joint Commonwealth, State and Territory funded program with the Commonwealth contributing 60% of the funds while the state contribute 40%. During 2004-05, AU$1.3B was provided nationally for the HACC program around Australia. The local programs that have developed are administered through all levels of government and community non-profit organizations. They provide a range of basic maintenance and support services to older people as well as people of all ages with a disability and their carers. This program aims to enhance independence and prevent premature institutionalization and includes, home nursing services, delivered meals, home help, home maintenance and modification services, transport and shopping assistance, allied health services, home- and center- based respite care [25].

The development of respite care services, and the introduction of the Community Aged Care Packages through Department of Health funding in the 1990's further supported the growth of community based care [7]. In 2001/02 the Commonwealth Government established the Extended Aged Care at Home (EACH) program for people in their own homes. These packages provide some funding for home modifications.

5. Service Responses

The following initiatives are nation wide services which address the home modifications needs of older people and people with a disability of any age

5.1. Carelink

Older people, people with disabilities and those who provide care are able to access free and confidential information on community aged care, disability and other support services available locally, interstate or anywhere within Australia through Carelink. Carelink is a nationwide network established by the Commonwealth in 2001. Consumers can access information via one of the 65 'walk in' shop fronts, calling a Freecall™ number or searching on their website www.commcarelink.health.gov.au.

5.2. Home and Community Care

The bulk of home and community based services for older people are provided under the auspices of this program. As one of many services provided under HACC, home maintenance and modification services received by consumers aged 65 in 2001-02 represented a small proportion of all service types: 14.4% and 3.1% respectively [7].

To be eligible for these services the person must be over 60 years, or any age with a disability and be a home owner or live in private rental housing. Many users pay a contribution towards the provisions of services, however in cases of financial difficulty, the provider is obliged to reduce or waive charges [7]. Individuals are not means tested for this service. Whilst HACC provides guidelines for service delivery, little is known about the criteria used for prioritizing or approving modifications and establishing user charges as there is no national data available [7]. It is known, however that these vary significantly among services within and between states. It is also evident that the coverage of service in the States and Territories is not complete, resulting in gaps in service. As well, there are inconsistent levels of capping on the home modification funding per individual around the States/Territories.

5.3. Departments of Housing

The States and Territories have a range of housing and housing related schemes funded through the CSHA. According to Bridge [10], these differ markedly and include schemes for public housing, community housing, loans for home purchase and rental assistance. Several state/territory governments have funded innovative responses to try and address the housing needs of older people and people with disabilities. These include construction of accommodation using principles of universal and adaptable design and provision of home modification programs to adapt existing public housing stock to meet the needs of this population where possible. Budgets around the various States and Territories range from AU$200K to AU$20M for home modifications, and from AU$0 to AU$137M for Capital Works (new construction and purchase of stock from the private market). Gaps still exist with respect to appropriate service provision to this population and also the indigenous communities.

5.4. Department of Veteran's Affairs

The Veterans' Affairs portfolio is responsible for carrying out Government policy and implementing programs to fulfill Australia's obligations to veterans and their dependants as well as providing compensation claims management service to current and former members of the Australian Defense Force. This Department provides assistance in the form of income support, compensation, care and commemoration programs for more than half a million veterans and their widows, widowers and dependants.

Veterans can access the Home Maintenance Helpline that provides property maintenance advice, or be referred to a reliable tradesperson for advice on home inspections, to identify current or possible future maintenance problems or HomeCare for home and garden maintenance for safety. HomeFront provides an annual home audit to make the homes of eligible veterans and war widows safer from falls and accident hazards. A free HomeFront assessment is available each calendar year and the Department makes a financial contribution towards the cost of recommended items and modifications. Minor and major Home Modifications are also provided to eligible veterans when problems are assessed as being related to war injury. A Home Support Loan is also available to eligible veterans, widows and widowers to assist with the cost of maintenance and modifications to their own homes, and other housing-related purposes that encourage independent living. The maximum loan is AU$10,000 (minimum drawing of AU$1,000) at a capped interest rate. To be eligible for these services the person must be a repatriation health card holder (gold and white) for specific conditions or with a defined clinical need. The person must also be the home owner or a long term private rental tenant. Veterans and war widows are required to make a co-payment for services.

During 2001-02, 49,965 people received services through Veterans' Home Care. Safety related maintenance was the second most commonly provided service, being provided to 36% of consumers. However this service averaged the least time, being 2 hours and 10 minutes per client for the year [7]. Home and garden maintenance constituted 29% of services offered in 2002 [6]. Veterans can also access different services from both the Veteran's Home Care program and the HACC funded programs. The Home Front program is not available in every State/Territory and its funding differs across Australia.

6. Specific Initiatives:

6.1. Smart Housing

Around Australia, there are several States/Territories that provide products to people in the private market (owners and renters) as well as to consumers in State owned public housing. In recognition of the lack of adequate accessible housing and home modification services in the private housing sector, the Queensland Department of Housing, under their Smart Housing Initiative, have introduced a range of strategies to try and both promote the development of housing that is socially, environmentally and economically sustainable and address the need for accessible housing in the private housing system. The Smart Housing Initiative incorporates the principles of universal design to integrate features that ensure a flexibility of use for people of varying abilities at different stages in their lives. Universal design is an approach to building homes that meet the needs of people across a range of ability and ages without the need for specialized design [21, 27].

6.2. Home Access and Home Loan Grant

As well as encouraging design initiatives for private housing providers the Queensland Department of Housing Smart Housing Initiative includes the Home Access Strategy, which aims to assist and empower individuals whose home environment places restrictions upon their ability to undertake usual day-to-day activities. This initiative has introduced a home loan program to provide private home owners access to low interest loans to carry out major modifications to their homes. This loan is between the value of AU$5K and AU$30K and is fixed at 4% per annum for a term of up to 30 years. The loan is being piloted in one region and it is anticipated that it will be made a statewide program in 2006-07. In addition, a grant for up to AU$10,000 is also available for people who have a Department of Housing home loan to assist with the modification of the home environment for people with a disability.

6.3. Home Assist Secure

Home Assist Secure is another initiative of the Queensland Department of Housing for private home owners or private renters who are aged 60 years and over, or who may be of any age with a disability. Recipients of this service must be receiving an Australian Commonwealth Government pension or benefit; and should not have other services or help available to assist them in the home, such as Home and Community Care, Veterans' Affairs or friends. Home Assist Secure provides free information, referrals and subsidized assistance to eligible consumers, such as: information and referrals about home maintenance, repairs, minor modifications and home security, including assistance with employing trades people, contracting experts or in planning future work; and inspections of the home to help people decide on security related repairs and installations. Staff trained by the Queensland Police Service conduct the inspections and can also provide information about personal security. Individuals can obtain subsidized assistance with minor home maintenance, repairs, modifications and security that relate to health, safety and security. There are 41 services in Queensland and modifications completed are generally up to the value of AU$1,000. There does not appear to be any other State or Territory Department of Housing in Australia that provides this type of service.

6.4. Home Renovation Grant

In Victoria, the Department of Human Services has developed a home renovation service whereby a loan of AU$25K and a grant of AU$5K is available to assist people over the age of 60, and individuals with disabilities or their carers, to modify their homes. They have teamed with Archicentre, to deliver this product. Archicentre is the building advisory service of the Royal Australian Institute of Architects. It offers architectural services and free technical advice to home buyers, new home builders and renovators. It provides a role in assessing homes and providing technical advice to people who wish to undertake home modifications to their premises.

6.5. Minor Modification Programs

There is a range of government and community agencies that provide minor modifications to individuals which are specific to the various states and territories around Australia. While funding is largely provided by the state governments, a number of the services are supported by not-for-profit organizations. These services are generally available to people in receipt of benefit cards that, in some cases, are required to pay for part of the cost of the modifications.

7. Outcomes

The success of the legislation, policies and services is determined by consumers throughout Australia achieving equal access to home modification and maintenance services. We also need to be certain that older people and people with disabilities are receiving the services they require to remain living in the community. Finally, we need to ascertain whether the home modification services are providing consumers with the outcomes they seek.

7.1. Do consumers have equal access to Home Modification Services?

There are approximately 3,500 HACC service delivery outlets across Australia, some of which are part of large organizations while others are small stand alone agencies staffed by one or two persons [1]. It is difficult to identify outcomes in community services due to the diverse client mix that is supported by various formal and informal supports. In addition there is a complex matrix of services, ranging from small agencies delivering single units of service to larger organizations providing a variety of maintenance, home modification and support services.

In an effort to monitor the accessibility and quality of HACC services the HACC Minimum Data Set (MDS) was developed. Originally commissioned in 1997, data collection began in January 2001. All service providers throughout Australia receiving funding via HACC are required to collect and report data. This data collection serves direct service planning and development. While HACC MDS contributes to program planning, monitoring and evaluation, it is important that it is seen as only one of several mechanisms which provide information for these purposes [1].

The HACC MDS is designed to be client centered and focuses on output/outcomes rather than processes. It records data about individual consumers, their circumstances and the types and level of assistance agencies provide to them individually. The data is collected on an ongoing basis rather than over a sample period and is aggregated for transmission in a quarterly collection cycle.

HACC aims to provide equitable services to people throughout Australia. Overall approx 20.6% of the total Australian population 65 years and over received HACC services during 2002-03. With rates of disability within this age group being 40% or more, it is evident that HACC services are reaching a good proportion of the population in need. The majority (92.4%) of service recipients were on some form of pension which indicates that whilst HACC is providing much needed services to older people with lower incomes, those with middle and higher incomes may not have access to information or services which can support them to age in place successfully. The majority of service recipients reported living in a private residence which they own or are purchasing (73%) while the remaining were in public (9.3%) or private (8.2%) rental accommodation. This data highlights the inequity experienced by people in rental accommodation. Whilst this is a small proportion of the older population it is likely that they are a venerable group with similar, if not greater service needs.

Rates of home modifications were similar in the homes of people who either owned their home (13.9%) or were boarders (14.6) or lived rent free (13.7%). However home modifications are less common (8%) in the homes of renters [7]. Recent data indicates that 59.6% of HACC consumers resided within the major cities, 25.1% in inner regional, 13% outer regional, 1.6% remote and .7% very remote [9]. These figures reflect the distribution of the Australian population between urban and regional areas which suggests that there is good coverage of services. However unofficial feedback suggests that service delivery is a "postcode lottery." It has been suggested that people living in rural and remote locations are frequently disadvantaged by the absence of services and personnel in their districts.

All HACC-funded agencies are currently undergoing external appraisal using the HACC National Service Standards Instrument developed at end of 2003-04, which also includes a Consumer Survey [7]. This will assess services provided against HACC standards.

7.2. Are consumers receiving the amount of support they require?

More specifically during 2003-04, there were 21,979 home modifications provided to HACC eligible consumers and 95,736 (13.5%) HACC consumers received a home maintenance service. This figure did not vary significantly from the previous year [9].

On average, 8 hours of home maintenance was provided to each HACC client over 2003-04. Data from the Disability, Aging and Carer Survey (DACS) 1998 indicates that only a small proportion of older people use government services (42.5/1000) compared to private home maintenance services (234.5/1000). Of concern is that the number of older people who indicated they had a need for home maintenance services was double that of those who were currently accessing government or private services [3].

Home modifications were provided to 21,979 (3%) HACC consumers with an average of AU$328 being spent per client per modification. Given the large percentage of older people who experience restrictions in core activities, it is surprising that only 3% of consumers received home modification services. It was reported by Bridge & Gopalan [10] that 10% of people aged over 65 years had to move in the five years prior to 1998 "due to 'profound' or 'severe' activity restriction caused by frailty or disability" (12). For people over 85, the likelihood of having moved was reported to be even higher [1, 5]. This discrepancy between the high rate of moving and low rate of HACC funded home modifications suggests that the home modification needs of older Australians is not being adequately met [10].

HACC MDS data reveals that the majority of home maintenance services (77%) and home modification services (76.5%) are provided to people over 70 years (see Table 1). The average cost of modifications were AU$224.40 for people over 75, AU$355.90 for people aged 65-69 and AU$730.90 for people less than 64 years.

Table 1. Home maintenance and modification services received by age

	0-64 years	65-69 years	70+ years	Total
Number of consumers				
Home Maintenance	14,401 (15)	7,603 (8)	73,732 (77)	95,736
Home Modifications	3,522 (16)	1,647(7.5)	16,810 (76.5)	21,979
Average service per client				
Home Maintenance *Hours*	11.8	7.4	7.3	8
Home Modifications *AU$*	730.9	355.9	241.4	328.4

For some people, access to home repair and modification services remains difficult. These rates appear to be low compared with the percentage of people who use aids. Usage rates for aids ranges from 87.0 % and 87.3% for people with profound and severe restrictions to 75.6% and 76.9% for people with moderate and mild restrictions. Home modifications are highest for older people (16.3%) and 0-14 years (11.1%) with other age groups ranging form 6.7% (15-29 years) to 8.1% (30-44years) and 8.2% (45-64 years) [7].

7.3. Are home modifications providing consumers with the outcomes they seek?

There has been limited investigation into the impact of home modifications on the health and independence of older people and people with disabilities in Australia. Studies in Australia on the impact of hazards in the home [12, 13, 23, 24] and modifications on falls in older people [15, 16, 25, 28, 29, 32] support the findings of studies in other countries. A direct relationship has yet to be established between environmental hazards in the home and the incidence of falls. When audit tools take into account the function of the individual within their home, rather than their environment in isolation, there is a stronger relationship. Similarly, home modifications have not been found to independently reduce falls risk. However, in combination with other interventions, home modifications contribute to a reduction in falls. In particular, home modifications provided in combination with a comprehensive home visit significantly reduced the risk of falling for frail older people who have previously fallen [14, 15].

Although a number of small unpublished studies have been undertaken in various services to identify the outcomes of home modifications, there has not been any systematic investigation into the impact on home modifications on the safety, independence, activity participation or health and well being of older Australians. A small study was undertaken by Veteran Affairs in 1996 [35] on 71 people who received a major modification. Yates & Knights found that the modifications reduced pain, increased community access, decreased anxiety, reduced physical assistance required, improved self esteem, reduced fear of performing activities, increased privacy in performing self care tasks, increased activity levels and decreased use of formal supports [35].

A study undertaken in 2002 by the Queensland Department of Housing on their home modification program, found that the majority of people reported moderate to extreme satisfaction with the completed modifications and felt that the changes had a positive impact on their safety, independence and quality of life. This study did, however, identify a number of issues that service providers need to be aware of, namely that the clients often have different priorities than the provider; modifications were perceived to have both positive and negative impacts; work was frequently not carried out as recommended; family dynamics and social circumstances can be impacted on by environmental modifications; and half the sample required further modifications that may have been unreported had a revisit not occurred [31].

A further qualitative study by Tanner in 2004 [30] also explored the impact of home modifications on the meaning of home for older people residing in public housing. This investigation found that home modifications have the potential to enhance the experience of home as a place of significant and unique personal and social meaning for older people. The study also found that the design of modifications, and other aspects of service delivery, supports a functionalist and bureaucratic approach that views the home as merely a physical environment or commodity. This approach can erode the meaning of home for the individual and diminish the effectiveness of home modifications.

8. Conclusion

This paper has reviewed the development of policies, funding and services in relation to the various demographic, social, and cultural issues that have arisen over time with the Australian population. It has detailed the legislative and policy responses which promote community living and the services which enable older people and people with disabilities to continue to live independently in their own homes. While current services are affordable and accessible to Australians who require support, further research is needed to determine the range of services and outcomes consumers seek.

References

[1] ABS. (1999). *Australian Social Trends 1999: Housing- Housing Assistance: Home Care, Hostels & Nursing Homes.* Canberra, Australia: Australian Bureau of Statistics.

[2] ABS. (2001). *Census of Population and Housing: Ageing in Australia 2001* (2048.0). Canberra: Australian Bureau of Statistics.
[3] ABS. (2003a). *Disability, Ageing and Carers, Australia.* (4430.0). Canberra, ACT.: Australian Bureau of Statistics.
[4] ABS. (2003b). *Population Projections Australia: 2002- 2101.* Canberra: Australian Bureau of Statistics.
[5] ABS. (2005). *Australian Social Trends* (4102.0). Canberra, ACT.: Australian Bureau of Statistics.
[6] AIHW. (2002). *Extended Aged Care at Home Census 2002.* Canberra, ACT.: Australian Institute of Health and Welfare.
[7] AIHW. (2003). *Australia's Welfare 2003.* Canberra Australia: Australian Institute of Health and Welfare.
[8] Andrews, K. (2002). *National Strategy for an Ageing Australia: an older Australia, challenges and opportunities for all.* Canberra: Department of Health and Ageing, Commonwealth, Government of Australia.
[9] Australian Government Department of Health and Ageing (2004) Home and Community Care Program Minimum Data Set 2003-2004 *Annual Bulletin.* Retrieved 28th September 2005 from www.health.gov.au/internet/wcms/Publishing.nsf/Content/hacc-pub_mds_sb.htm
[10] Bridge, C & Gopalan, P. (2005) Retrofitting, a response to lack of diversity: An analysis of community provider data, *National Housing Conference*, 26-28 October, Perth.
[11] Bridge, C., Parsons, A., Quine, S., & Kendig, H. (2002). *Housing and care for older and younger adults with disabilities : Positioning Paper.* Sydney Australia.: Australian Housing and Urban Research Institute.
[12] Carter, S. E., Campbell, E. M., Sanson Fisher, R. W., & Gillespie, W. J. (2000). Accidents in older people living at home: a community-based study assessing prevalence, type, location and injuries. *Australian and New Zealand Journal of Public Health*, 24(6), 633-636.
[13] Clemson, L., Cumming, R. G., & Roland, M. (1996). Case-control study of hazards in the home and risk of falls and hip fractures. *Age and Ageing*, 25(2), 97-101.
[14] Close, J., Ellis, M., Hooper, R., Glucksman, E, Jackson, S., & Swift, C. (1999). Prevention of falls in the elderly trial (PROFET): a randomised controlled trial. *Lancet*, 353(9147), 93-97.
[15] Cumming, R. G., Thomas, M., Szonyi, G., Salkeld, G., O'Neill, E., Westbury, C., & Frampton, G. (1999). Home visits by an occupational therapist for assessment and modification of environmental hazards: a randomized trial of falls prevention. *Journal of the American Geriatrics Society*, 47(12), 1397-1402.
[16] Day, L., Fildes, B., Gordon, I., Fitzharris, M., Flamer, H., & Lord, S. (2002). Randomised factorial trial of falls prevention among older people living in their own homes. *BMJ Clinical Research ed,* 325(7356), 128.
[17] Duncan, R. (1998). Funding, Financing and other resources for Home Modifications. *Technology and Disability, 8*, 37-50.
[18] Fange, A., & Iwarsson, S. (2005). Changes in ADL Dependence and Aspects of Usability Following Housing Adaptation - A Longitudinal Perspective. *The American Journal of Occupational Therapy, 59*(3), 296-304.
[19] Faulkner, D., & Bennett, K. (2002). *Linkages among housing assistance, residential (re) location and the use of community health and social care by old-old adults: shelter and non-shelter implications for housing policy development.* Sydney, Australia: Australian Housing and Urban Research Institute.
[20] Gray, L. (2001). *Two Year Review of Aged Care Reforms.* Canberra ACT: Department of Health and Aged Care.
[21] Heumann, L. F., & Boldy, D. P. (Eds.). (1993). *Aging in Place with Dignity: International Solutions Relating to the Low Income and Frail Elderly.* Westport CT.: Praeger Publishers.
[22] Mace, R. L. (1998). Universal Design in Housing. *Assistive Technology, 10*, 21 -28.
[23] Mackenzie, L., Byles, J., & Higginbotham, N. (2002). A prospective community-based study of falls among older people in Australia: Frequency, circumstances, and consequences. *OTJR Occupation Participation and Health*, 22(4), 143-152.
[24] McLean, D., & Lord, S. (1996). Falling in older people at home: transfer limitations and environmental risk factors. *Australian Occupational Therapy Journal*, 43(1), 13-18.
[25] National Program Guidelines for the Home and Community Care Program, 2002
Peel, N., Steinberg, M., & Williams, G. (2000). Home safety assessment in the prevention of falls among older people. *Australian and New Zealand Journal of Public Health*, 24(5), 536-539.
[26] Pynoos, J. (1993). Toward a national policy on home modifications. *Technology and Disability*(2), 1-8.

[27] Sanford, J. A., Follette Story, M., & Tingholz, D. (1998). Consumer participation to inform universal design. *Technology and Disability, 9*, 149 -162.

[28] Steinberg, M., Cartwright, C., Peel, N., & Williams, G. (2000). A sustainable programme to prevent falls and near falls in community dwelling older people: results of a randomised trial. *Journal of Epidemiology and Community Health,* 54(3), 227-232.

[29] Stevens, M., Holman, C. D., Bennett, N., & de Klerk, N. (2001). Preventing falls in older people: outcome evaluation of a randomized controlled trial. *Journal of the American Geriatrics Society*, 49(11), 1448-1455.

[30] Tanner, B (2004) *The Impact of Home Modifications on the Meaning of Home for Older People Living in the Community*, Unpublished Masters Thesis, The University of Queensland, Brisbane

[31] Tanner, B. & Middleton, K. (2002) Home Modification: How well are we doing it? Australian Association of Occupational Therapists Queensland State Conference for Occupational Therapists, 19th -21st September, Townsville.

[32] Thompson, P. G. (1996). Preventing falls in the elderly at home: a community-based program. *Medical Journal of Australia*, 164(9), 530-532.

[33] Tinker, A. (1999) Ageing in Place: What Can We Learn From Each Other, *The Sixth F.Oswald Barnett Oration*, 9th September 1999, Melbourne.

[34] WHO. (2001). *ICIDH-2: International Classification of Functioning and Disability.* Geneva: World Health Organization.

[35] Yates, S & Knights, K Assessing the outcomes of high cost home modifications, unpublished report, Department of Veteran Affairs, Brisbane.

Promoting Independence for Older Persons with Disabilities
W.C. Mann and A. Helal (Eds.)
IOS Press, 2006

Standing Up: A Systematic Review of Grabrail Orientations

H. SETON[a,1], C. BRIDGE[a]
[a]*School of Occupation and Leisure Sciences, Faculty of Health Sciences, University of Sydney, Australia*

Abstract. Performing a sit to stand transfer is a prerequisite for many activities of daily living. In fact, most people perform this transfer many times each day; when getting out of bed, after sitting at the table for a meal and during toileting. However, this transfer has been defined as one of the most biomechanically difficult functional tasks, which only becomes more difficult as people age [21]. To aid this transfer, particularly for older people performing a toilet sit to stand transfer, equipment or home modifications are generally prescribed. The home modifications commonly consist of the installation of a grabrail. However, there remains much debate among therapists worldwide as to the correct positioning and orientation for grabrails. This study aims to provide a comprehensive overview of the existing literature to identify the effects of grabrail orientation on the body and areas which require further research. To complete this research project a systematic review protocol was adopted. This is a rigorous process which ensures that all relevant and available literature on a given topic is located, reviewed and analysed. A specific search strategy was developed to ensure a comprehensive search of all data sources was completed. The data included in this review was obtained from a variety of sources including electronic databases, the World Wide Web and legislation and regulatory documents. A strict inclusion and exclusion criteria were developed to ensure only the most important and relevant information was included in this review. A total of 27 articles and 15 national and international legislation and regulatory documents were located and included in this systematic review. A majority of the research located was completed in the United States of America and Australia. Many of the articles were biomechanically oriented and focused on the older population, who more regularly use grabrails. All of the articles included in this systematic review agreed that some form of arm support, be it grabrails or armrests, provided support to the body while performing a sit to stand transfer. However, no clear recommendations could be made on which orientation of grabrail assists the person without causing undue stress. From the results, specific biomechanical stresses were identified for each grabrail orientation. Further research is required in this area to develop improved guidelines for therapists, policy makers, home modification providers and consumers alike.

Keywords. Grabrail, transfer, activities of daily living, home modifications

Introduction:

Australia's population is ageing. By 2051 the projected percentage of our population over the age of 65 will be between 27% and 30% [3]. This will have risen from the current situation where older people comprise just under 13% of the population [4]. The increase in the older population is due primarily to an increased life expectancy in combination with a decreased fertility rate. Concurrent with the ageing process, bodily changes may affect an older person's functional performance such as mobility and self care.

For example, the ageing process has been linked to a generalized decrease in muscle strength and joint range of motion, especially at the hip, knee and spine, as well as difficulties with proprioception and balance which in turn affects performance during a sit to stand transfer [1, 15]. Additionally, older people typically experience a generalized slowing of many of the body systems including the nervous, sensory and cognitive systems [10, 14, 20]. As the nervous system overarches all other body systems, a person may become slower to react to sensory stimuli; as a result generalized slowing of motor responses and cognitive processes may also be evident. Consequently the process of ageing affects how an older person manages a sit to stand transfer.

Sanford, Arch, & Megrew [23] maintain that grabrail provision based on a thorough assessment of the person and their environment can provide the person with an increased sense of safety and greater independence. This is unsurprising given that environmental hazards have been found to be a contributing factor in most falls around the home, including in the bathroom and toilet [9]. Typically during the home visit and/or functional assessment the hazards specific to the individual and their environment are identified and steps are then taken to reduce any hazards identified. Consequently it is fairly common for assistive devices such as grabrails to be recommended and installed in the bathroom [11, 25, 28]. Thus grabrail prescription and installation has the potential to minimise the effects that disability or old age have on the performance of the sit to stand transfer.

The primary purpose of the majority of grabrails installed in the bathroom and toilet is to assist a difficult transfer in a wet environment. Provision of grabrails at toilets is often seen as a prerequisite for safe and independent toileting, particularly in the older population [23]. Therefore it is essential that older people have access to correctly installed and positioned grabrails which will assist with the sit to stand transfer. Along with the high installation rate these assistive devices have a high usage and satisfaction rate [2, 11, 12, 25, 26, 28].

Regardless of the frequency of prescription of grabrails, many issues arise concerning positioning and orientation of the grabrail. Much of the research which has been completed focuses on the rate of prescription and rate of use rather than the specifics of orientation of the grabrail. Clemson and Martin [11] assessed 144 older participants regarding the use and effectiveness of rails in the bathroom and toilet and found that even though most people used the rails installed next to their toilets some were dissatisfied with the placement and orientation. However, little is known how the use of each grabrail orientation affects the body during a sit to stand transfer.

The sit to stand transfer involves many specific and difficult movements, such as developing adequate torque at the knee and hip joints, in conjunction with coordination of spatial and temporal motion of the body segments [5]. The successful completion of a sit to stand transfer also depends on the range of motion of the joints and the forces placed on the body. Through these movements the body's center of mass moves from an intrinsically stable three point support during sitting to a dynamically stable two point support when standing [7, 21].

The way a sit to stand transfer is performed changes as a person ages. Many of these changes relate to a decrease in muscle strength, such as the development of adequate torque and controlling momentum [1, 6, 28]. Chair rise strategy also changes along with the time taken to rise successfully [1]. The consistency of the movements among the older population also decreases, which provides a signal to the changes that may be occurring throughout the transfer. To assist with this transfer grabrails may be prescribed. The effect that a grabrail and its orientation may have on the body has yet to be clearly defined. This paper aims to compare and collate all this information to provide a comprehensive outline of the effects of grabrail orientation on the body.

1. Methodology

A systematic review, guided by the *Protocol guidelines for systematic reviews of home modification information to inform best practice* [8] developed by the Home Modification and Maintenance Information Clearinghouse was used to complete this study. Specific search terms were identified from the research question and comprehensive literature review and were used to search for appropriate material on electronic databases and the World Wide Web. Table 1 contains the search terms, including those that were truncated.

Table 1. Search Terms

Environment	Person	Activity
Grabrail*	Older population*	Sit to stand transfer*
Grab rail*	Older people*	Sit to stand*
Grab bar*	Aging	Sitting to standing*
Rail*	Age*	
Grab-rail*	Elderly*	
Handrail*	Senior*	
Toilet		
Lavatory		
Bathroom		
Commode		
Horizontal		
Vertical		

A wide variety of electronic databases were selected to ensure a comprehensive search was undertaken and all articles of relevance were located. A structured search strategy was developed which combined the above search terms. The following is a list of all areas searched.

- HMM Info Library
- Ageline
- AMED (Allied and Complementary Medicine)
- AMI: Australasian Medical Index
- ARCH: Australian Architecture Database
- AVE: Avery Index to Architectural Periodicals
- CINAHL (Nursing and Allied Health)
- Compendex Plus
- Current Contents
- Dissertation abstracts
- Expanded Academic Index ASAP
- Medline
- OSH-ROM
- ProQuest 5000

- PsycINFO
- PubMed
- Science Direct
- University of Sydney Theses
- Web of Science
- WWW via the Google and Google Scholar Search engine
- Legislative and Regulatory Documents

Specific inclusion and exclusion criteria were developed to ensure only the most relevant articles were included in the review. Material was included if it was (a) accessible through the University of Sydney Library network or the World Wide Web, (b) written in English, (c) a human study and (d) printed after 1950 due to the changes in the home modification industry and the understanding of biomechanics. Materials which did meet the inclusion criteria or were whole of subject books, editorials or conference papers were not included in the review. Figure 1 illustrates the search process and the final number of articles included in this study.

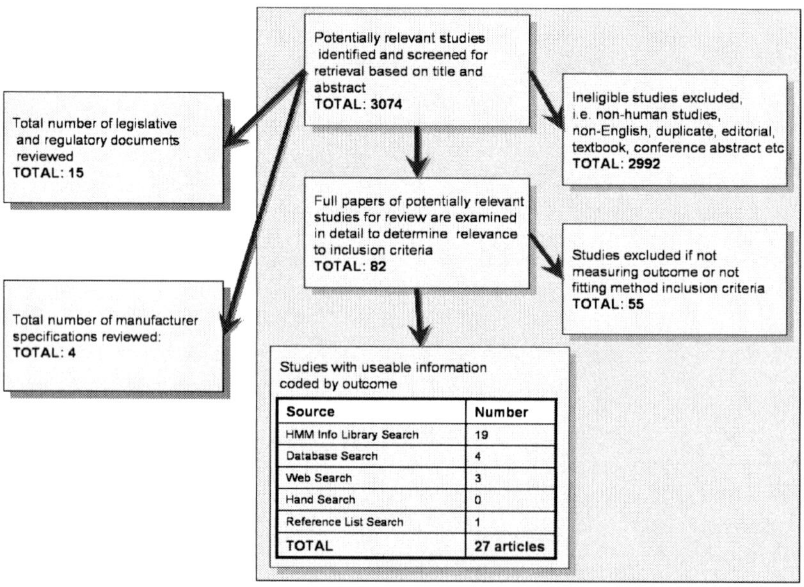

Figure 1: Search process and number of articles included during searching

2. Results:

The material included in this study was located from the HMM Info Library, Ageline, AMED and AMI databases as well as the World Wide Web. This study reviewed twenty seven articles, fifteen legislation documents and four manufacturer specifications. The articles located covered a span of fifteen years, with the earliest article being published in 1990. The majority of the articles were published in the United States of America, followed by Australia. Figure 2 shows the nationality of the articles reviewed.

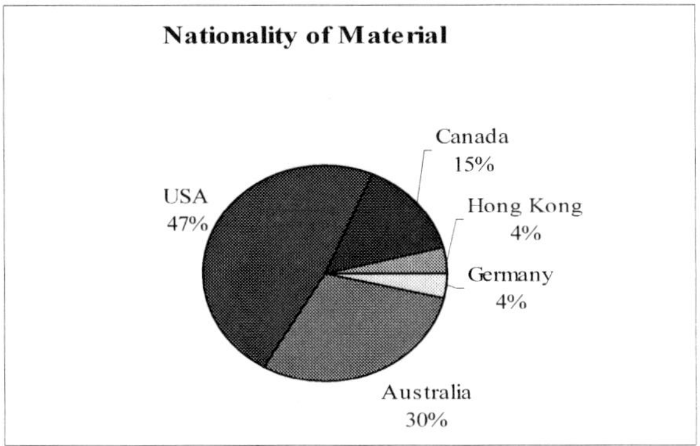

Figure 2: Nationality of Material

Over half the studies included in this review were completed using a quasi-experimental methodology. This was the highest form of research evidence located. No systematic reviews or randomised control trials were located. Expert opinion comprised a third of the articles, with both case study and anecdotal evidence each comprising 4% of the articles. Figure 3 illustrates the methodology types of the included articles.

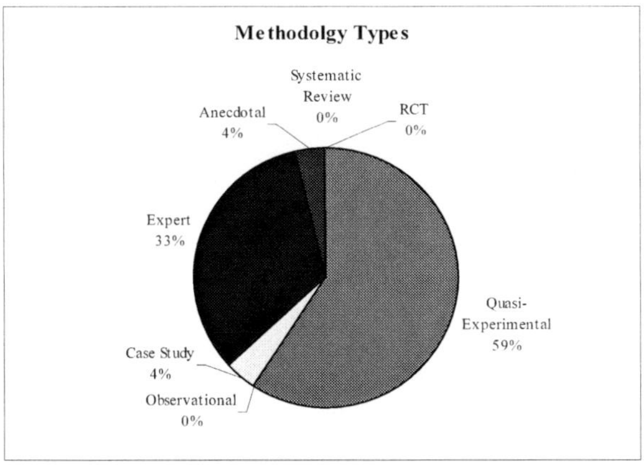

Figure 3: Methodology Types

The variables from each included article were defined by activity, person or environment. By encoding the variables a judgement regarding the relevance of the article to this study could be made. In addition, the important elements from each article could be recorded quickly. Tables 2, 3 and 4 outline the variables for each and demonstrate how many times each was located in the included articles

Table 2: Activity Variables

Activity Variable	Number of Times Recorded
Sit to Stand Toilet	14
Sit to Stand Other (e.g. chair)	9
Sit to Stand Incident (e.g. fall)	0

Table 3: Person Variables

Person Variable	Number of Times Recorded
Older Healthy	16
Older Other (e.g. arthritis)	3
All Ages	7

Table 4: Environment Variables

Environment Variable	Number of Times Recorded
Vertical Grabrail	13
Horizontal Grabrail	13
Grabrail Other (e.g. Angled)	14
Armrest	5

The information collected from the articles provided valuable insight into how a grabrail and varying orientations may affect the body, particularly that of an older person, when used to assist with the sit to stand transfer. The following discussion will center on the impact that the horizontal and vertical grabrails have on the body.

3. Discussion

Grabrail orientation can have a profound affect on the body of an older person. Men and women have individual anthropometric dimensions, such as height, along with different requirements [7]. Because of these differences a single grabrail orientation will provide a different level of assistance to each person. However, it has been found that orientation can influence the mechanics of a sit to stand transfer for able-bodied people [16]. The following paragraphs provide an overview of how a grabrail and the differing orientations may affect the body, including peak joint angles, range of motion, forces and torque. It will be necessary to remember that not all people will experience all changes, and the changes experienced will be in varying degrees.

3.1. Peak Angles

Generally the peak joint angles are reduced when using a grabrail [16]. However, only a small number of articles discuss the change in joint angles. O'Meara [16] discussed the specific joints in which changes occur. With a single laterally placed (to the right of the participant) grabrail, changes were seen in the right ankle, left hip, the lumbar spine and the neck [17]. However, changes were different depending on the orientation of the grabrail. With the use of a vertical grabrail greater reductions are seen in the angle of the neck and the right ankle, where a greater reduction in the left hip is seen with the use of a horizontal grabrail [16].

In two vertical grabrail studies peak joint angles were also discussed [18, 22]. Agreement between the reduction in the hip peak joint angle is noted between these studies and the above study by O'Meara [16]. However, in these studies no specific hip (left or right) is noted [18, 22]. In addition, the knee flexion joint angle was noted to reduce with the use of a vertical grabrail. However, Ongley [18] did not find this change to be statistically significant, compared to Roland [22] who found a significant reduction in the knee flexion angle. These changes in the peak joint angle will vary from person to person. Both these studies had comparable participant groups of older healthy women and the methodology was very similar. Therefore it is unclear why a difference was found in the knee joint peak angles. However, all other joint angles were found to have changed when a grabrail, particularly a vertical grabrail, was used.

3.2. Range Of Motion

The range of motion of the joints in both the upper and lower limbs is affected when using a grabrail. Most researchers agreed that with the use of a grabrail, either horizontal or vertical, that the range of motion at the hip joint is reduced [13, 16, 18, 22]. O'Meara [16] found that a vertical grabrail was best at reducing the range of motion in the hip closest to the grabrail, where the horizontal grabrail reduced the range of motion in the other hip.

In addition a reduction of range of motion was also noted in the knee [16, 18, 22]. O'Meara [16] found that the vertical grabrail was best at reducing the range of motion in both knees. It was noted by Roland [22] that those participants who relied on the grabrail more heavily had a larger reduction. However, Ongley [18] found the change in the knee to be slight, where McDonald [13] found no change when using a grabrail. It is unclear as to why a difference was found between these studies. Each used a comparable sample of healthy older people, excluding McDonald [13] who had older participants with arthritis. Each also used very similar study designs including force plates and motion analysis systems. Having such similar studies highlights the variations in effect that a grabrail can have on the body.

A similar pattern to the knee range of motion was also observed at the ankle. A reduction in the required range of motion of the ankle has been shown to occur with grabrail use [16, 18]. O'Meara [16] stated that the vertical grabrail orientation was best at reducing the range of motion of the ankle closest to the grabrail. Again, McDonald [13], in her study found no reduction in the range of motion required at the ankle. This again emphasises the variations that can exist between each user of a grabrail.

The influence on the range of motion of the upper limb has only been discussed by two studies [16, 19]. It was suggested that the grabrail orientation can influence the range of motion of the upper limb [16]. Each orientation places the arm in a different position, which causes the joints to move differently. However, very limited literature has been published on the biomechanics of the upper limb during an assisted sit to stand transfer. Packer et al [19] however does discuss the range of motion which the elbow and forearm moves through when using an armrest. The range of motion that the elbow moves through was found to be 77.1 degrees and the forearm through 24.4 degrees of motion [19]. This highlights an area which must be covered before any definite conclusions about the correct orientation can be made.

3.3. Forces

Forces which act on the body during the sit to stand transfer can vary greatly depending on the orientation and the support a person requires. It was shown that hand placement can determine how much force is placed through the body when using a grabrail [17]. Hand placement is influenced by the orientation of the grabrail. Therefore, the grabrail orientation can affect the forces on the body [17]. When using a vertical grabrail the largest grabrail force is found in the anterior-posterior direction, which suggests that the person is pulling posteriorly on the grabrail [22]. This is in contrast to the horizontal grabrail in which a person pushes down on the grabrail to assist with the transfer. The hand forces when using a horizontal assistance of an armrest, were found to be between 114.0 Newtons and 158.9 Newtons for both young and old participants [1]. However, when expressing this force as a ratio of body weight the older participants have significantly larger values [1]. Arm support is used to compensate for a reduction in leg and trunk strength. This demonstrates the reliance that older people place on arm assistance when completing this transfer.

An assisted sit to stand transfer has varying effects of the forces experienced at the lower extremity joints. Bahrami et al [5] found that the maximum forces in the lower extremity joints are significantly reduced at seat off when using strong arm support. However, a general pattern of an increase in the shear joint forces and a decrease in the compressive forces of the hip and knee has been demonstrated in other studies [13, 16, 18]. O'Meara [16] found that in this general pattern the changes in forces depended on the side of the body which the grabrail was placed. For example, with a grabrail placed on the right side the shear joint forces in the right ankle and knee increased. The right hip experienced no changes in shear joint force. The compressive forces in the right hip however did increase. The shear joint forces in the ankle, knee and hip on the left however, experienced a significant reduction [16]. The increase in the shear joint forces may prove to be a contraindication for grabrails for those people who have joint instability or conditions which affect the integrity of the joint itself. This should be kept in mind when prescribing a grabrail, despite the orientation.

3.4. Torque

Varying opinions regarding the relationship between torque and grabrail use have been discussed in the literature [5, 16, 24]. In the study by Bahrami and colleagues [5] it was noted that strong arm support reduces the maximum required torque of the lower extremities at seat off. However, Schultz et al [24] suggested that arm assistance is used more to gain postural stability rather than reducing the torque requirements at seat off. Despite this claim it is widely accepted that a reduction in joint torque occurs when using a grabrail by Schultz et al and other researchers [5, 13, 16, 18, 22, 24]. When studying the joint torque O'Meara [16] found that an asymmetric change occurs due to the unilateral nature of the assistance. This is an important fact when considering older people who may have one-sided weakness or joint pain. Ensuring safe and effective grabrails are installed which compliment the user must be a priority.

Schultz et al [24] found that the shoulder joint torque requirements increase when using a grabrail compared to not using a grabrail because larger push magnitudes are generated [24]. More surprisingly, they found that if the push direction was more vertical the required torque at the shoulder could be substantially reduced. However, these findings were achieved by using an armrest rather than a grabrail. The results relate most closely to a horizontal grabrail and findings such as these demonstrate that a wall mounted horizontal grabrail may produce large torque around the shoulder joint. There was no literature available which discussed the torque at the shoulder when using a vertical grabrail and the study by Schultz et al [24] was the only study found which discussed torque in relation to horizontal arm assistance. This highlights a rather large gap in the research which will need to be addressed in the near future.

The joint torque at the hip has been found to reduce with the use of a grabrail [5, 18, 22, 24]. The hip extension torque was found to be reduced significantly suggesting the use of a grabrail may relieve the muscular effort surrounding the hip during the extension phase of the transfer [18, 22] In addition the maximum hip flexion torque was found to slightly decreases when using a grabrail [18]. This torque can also be affected by the size and direction of assistance. A greater push magnitude can slightly reduce the hip torque while a vertical push direction substantially reduces the required hip torque [24]. The findings from each of these studies reflect both horizontal and vertical grabrail use. From the results it is assumed that both grabrail orientations reduce the required hip torque. However, without a study which directly compares the two, no judgement can be made as to the orientation which reduces torque most significantly.

Two opposite findings have been located regarding the knee joint torque during as assisted transfer. A majority of researchers found that both the knee extension and flexion torque decrease when using a grabrail [5, 13, 18, 24]. However, the knee extension torque significantly increased in all the participants in the study by Roland [22]. The participants, all older healthy women, experienced an increase in the required torque which indicates an increase in the stress on the knee joint and an increase in the required muscular effort. This study utilised a vertical grabrail, however, a vertical grabrail was also used in the studies by McDonald [13] and Ongley [18]. It is unclear to why there is such a difference in these results.

The results discussing the effect of a grabrail on the required ankle torque are varied. A general increase in the required ankle torque was found by two researchers who were using horizontal aids in their research [5, 24]. This is in contrast to research conducted with vertical grabrails which found a significant reduction in plantar flexion torque and a slight decrease in dorsiflexion torque [13, 18]. However, a third researcher also using a vertical grabrail found a significant increase in the required plantarflexion torque and a significant decrease in required dorsiflexion torque [22]. These results suggest that a horizontal grabrail may increase the required ankle torque where a vertical grabrail may decrease torque. In addition, the results from Roland [22] also suggest that a vertical grabrail may increase the torque in some people. This again highlights the need for further research in the area of the biomechanics of an assisted sit to stand transfer.

3.5. Asymmetry

When a grabrail is positioned laterally to a person, which is most always the case, an asymmetry in the motion of the sit to stand transfer occurs [16]. An asymmetric change is produced in the net joint forces and torque due the unilateral nature of the assistance [16]. For example increases in compressive forces of the right hip, the shear joint forces in the right ankle and shear joint forces in the right knee all occur with a grabrail placed on the right side of the body [16]. This occurrence should not be taken lightly, particularly with older people who may have one sided weakness, for example from a stroke. By considering this factor a grabrail, either horizontal or vertical, can be placed on the most appropriate side for a person to use without causing any undue stress or strain on already weakened muscles.

3.6. Postural Stability and Balance

A person's balance and postural stability during a toilet sit to stand transfer can be assisted when using a grabrail [27]. This assistance is particularly important when getting off the seat, which is one of the most unstable instances during the transfer [24]. When using grabrail assistance a person's center of mass is outside the base of support when getting off the seat [5]. This suggests that the arm support is used to increase balance and the person's ability to complete the sit to stand transfer. In addition, a vertical grabrail has been shown to assist in the stabilization phase of the transfer. The vertical grabrail provides a higher support for a person to hold until their body has stabilized before beginning their gait pattern [7]. This can be very important in preventing balance related falls in the toilet and bathroom. A horizontal grabrail does not provide as much assistance during this time as they are generally positioned to low to provide adequate support.

4. Conclusion

The findings of this systematic review provide a basis for understanding how grabrail orientation can affect the body. Both positive and negative effects occur. To ensure that the correct grabrail orientation is provided to the client these effects must be considered. For example if a person has arthritis which affects the ankle joint, a horizontal grabrail, which increases the required torque at the ankle joint, may not provide the best assistance without causing undue stress on the joint. So, before prescribing a grabrail orientation the client's personal circumstances and abilities must be considered; particularly until further biomechanical research can be conducted. Large gaps exist in the research regarding how a grabrail orientation can affect the body, particularly in terms of the upper limbs. This research must be conducted before further conclusions can be made regarding grabrail orientation.

5. Acknowledgements

The HMMinfo project team gratefully acknowledges the financial and other support received from the NSW Department of Ageing, Disability and Home Care (DADHC) and the Commonwealth Home and Community Care Program without which this work would not have been possible. The authors would also like to acknowledge the contribution of many experts from the Home Modification and Maintenance Services within NSW, Occupational Therapists and the grabrail industry who generously gave of their time and expertise, without them all sharing their ideas, perspectives and information this synthesis could not have been generated.

References:

[1] Alexander, N. B., Schultz, A. B., & Warwick, D. N. (1991). Rising from a Chair: Effects of Age and Functional Ability on Performance Biomechanics. Journal of Gerontology, 46(3), M91.

[2] Aminzadeh, F., & Edwards, N. (1998). Exploring Seniors' Views on the Use of Assistive Devices in Fall Prevention. [Article]. Public Health Nursing August, 15(4), 297-304.

[3] Australian Bureau of Statistics. (2003). Population projections: Australia 2002 - 2101. Canberra, Australia: Australian Bureau of Statistics.

[4] Australian Bureau of Statistics. (2005). Year book Australia: Population: Population size and growth. Australia: Australian Bureau of Statistics.

[5] Bahrami, F., Riener, R., Jabedar-Maralani, P., & Schmidt, G. (2000). Biomechanical analysis of sit-to-stand transfer in healthy and paraplegic subjects. Clinical Biomechanics, 15(2), 123-133.

[6] Beissner, K. L., Collins, J. E., & Holmes, H. (2000). Muscle force and range of motion as predictors of function in older adults. Physical Therapy, 80(6), 556 - 563.

[7] Bridge, C. (2003). Basic biomechanical and anatomical principles underpinning grabrail prescription for sit to stand transfers. Sydney, Australia: University of Sydney.
[8] Bridge, C., & Phibbs, P. (2003). Protocol guidelines for systematic reviews of home modification information to inform best practice. Sydney: University of Sydney, Faculty of Health Sciences and Architecture.
[9] Carter, S. E., Campbell, E. M., Sanson-Fisher, R. W., Redman, S., & Gillespie, W. J. (1997). Environmental hazards in the homes of older people. Age and Ageing, 26(3), 195.
[10] Carter, W. B., McKenna, M., Martin, M. L., & Andresen, E. M. (1989). Health education: Special issues for older adults. Patient Education and Counseling, 13, 117 - 131.
[11] Clemson, L., & Martin, R. (1996). Usage and effectiveness of rails, bathing and toileting aids. Occupational therapy in health care, 10(1), 41 - 59.
[12] Edwards, N. I., & Jones, D. A. (1998). Ownership and use of assistive devices amongst older people in the community. Age and Ageing, 27(4), 462.
[13] McDonald, G. (1997). An investigation into vertical grabrail use and grabrail height for older women with bilateral knee osteoarthritis. Unpublished Honours Thesis, University of Sydney, Sydney: Australia.
[14] McLean, D., & Lord, S. (1996). Falling in older people at home: Transfer limitations and environmental risk factors. Australian Occupational Therapy Journal, 43, 13 - 18.
[15] Millington, P. J., Myklebust, B. M., & Shambes, G. M. (1992). Biomechanical analysis of the sit-to-stand motion in elderly persons. Archives of physical and medical rehabilitation, 73(7), 609 - 617.
[16] O'Meara, D. M. (2003). Properties of manual support fixtures. Unpublished PhD Thesis, University of Sydney, Sydney: Australia.
[17] O'Meara, D. M., & Smith, R. M. (2005). Differences between grab rail position and orientation during the assisted sit-to-stand for able-bodied older adults. Journal of Applied Biomechanics, 21(1), 57 - 71.
[18] Ongley, J. (1999). An investigation of the sit-to-stand transfer in healthy older women when standing up from different toilet pan heights, with and without grabrail assistance., Unpublished Honours Thesis University of Sydney, Sydney: Australia.
[19] Packer, T. L., Wyss, U. P., & Costigan, P. A. (1993). Elbow kinematics during sit-to-stand and stand-to-sit movements. Clinical Biomechanics, 8, 322 - 328.
[20] Rice, F. P. (1986). Adult development and aging. Massachusetts, USA: Allyn and Bacon, Inc.
[21] Riley, P. O., Schenkman, M., Mann, R. W., & Hodge, W. A. (1991). Mechanics of a constrained chair rise. Journal of Biomechanics, 24(1), 77-85.
[22] Roland, M. (1996). Effectiveness of grabrails during sit to stand transfers. Unpublished Masters Thesis, University of Sydney, Sydney: Australia.
[23] Sanford, J. A., Arch, M., & Megrew, M. B. (1995). An evaluation of grab bars to meet the needs of elderly people. Assistive technology, 7, 36-47.
[24] Schultz, A. B., Alexander, N. B., & Ashton-Miller, J. A. (1992). Biomechanical analyses of rising from a chair. Journal of Biomechanics, 25(12), 1383 - 1391.
[25] Sonn, U., & Grimby, G. (1994). Assistive devices in an elderly population studies at 70 and 76 years of age. Disability and Rehabilitation, 16(2), 85 - 92.
[26] Stark, S. (2004). Removing Environmental Barriers in the Homes of Older Adults With Disabilities Improves Occupational Performance. OTJR, 24(1), 32 - 39.
[27] Tideiksaar, R. (1990). Environment adaptations to preserve balance and prevent falls. Topics in Geriatric Rehabilitation, 5(2), 78 - 84.
[28] Trickey, F., Maltais, D., Gosselin, C., & Robitaille, Y. (1993). Adapting older persons' homes to promote independence. Physical and occupational therapy in geriatrics, 12(1), 1-14.

Promoting Independence for Older Persons with Disabilities
W.C. Mann and A. Helal (Eds.)
IOS Press, 2006

Lighting Your Way into Home Modifications

M. PITCH[a,1], C. BRIDGE[a]
[a]*School of Occupation and Leisure Sciences, Faculty of Health Sciences, University of Sydney, Australia*

Abstract. Good quality lighting in the home can make the difference between seeing and not seeing for someone with vision impairment. This presentation will discuss a systematic review that investigated whether wayfinding light systems are capable of providing adequate illumination to enable safe and independent mobility. It will outline the research that is currently available on lighting for people with vision impairment and how this information can be used within the home modification industry.

Keywords. Home modifications, low vision, lighting, independent mobility

Introduction

This paper examines previous lighting research to try to answer two overarching questions as they relate to indoor mobility of persons with visual impairments. On one hand the issue of the range of illumination values suitable for ensuring safe and independent mobility within the home of an individual with vision impairment is examined. Second, the effectiveness of ambient lighting versus task lighting in providing this level of illumination is explored. The material currently available relevant to these questions is then analyzed to try to determine best practice guidance.

The systematic review methodology adopted to investigate the research questions involved searching electronic databases, grey literature, and legislation and manufactures specifications. In total 14 legislative and regulatory documents and 36 articles were identified that met all the inclusion criteria. Analysis of material showed that the majority of material located focused on changes associated with physiological vision impairment (81%) followed by discussion of illumination levels (72%).

As a result it appears that an ambient lighting system can enable safe movement through a building at levels of between 20 - 40 lux [37, 38, 41], while adequate illumination for task lighting, such as a wayfinding light systems can be as low as 0.05 - 1 lux [1, 43, 44]. This is because task lighting is able to create a contrast with the background environment emphasizing the pathway of travel

1. Background

This section sets out the four key variables relevant to understanding and analyzing lighting for people with vision impairment.

1.1. The human visual system is dependent on light

The visual system is vital for obtaining information about the environment and the individual's position within the environment [36]. This information plays a fundamental role in the activity of mobility, enabling individuals to orientate themselves, scan the environment for potential hazards and navigate their way through a safe pathway of travel [21].

Sight depends on the quality of light in the environment and this is evident in the number of physiological adaptations that attempt to make maximum use of the light available. For example, the iris controls the amount of light entering the eye and the cornea focuses the light onto the retina. Although the eye makes optimal use of the light it cannot compensate for a lack of light and in its absence, vision cannot occur [4]. Vision impairment is experienced when the eye is unable to process the light effectively (physiological vision impairment) or when light is of a poor quality (environmental vision impairment).

1.2. The activity of mobility

Vision is the primary sensory modality used for obtaining information about the environment to enable the safe performance of mobility [33]. Vision enables the individual to orientate themselves to the environment, preview the environment and visually validate their immediate space [47]. One of the most significant handicaps caused by vision impairment is the limit imposed on the ability to travel independently [18].

The activity of mobility enables movement from point A to point B allowing freedom and independence to explore the environment and perform essential daily activities [20]. A restriction in mobility can reduce an individual's independence and they can become more dependent on others to perform their basic day-to-day activities; this can severely reduce their quality of life [29].

1.3. The hallway environment

The environment can impact the performance of safe mobility, particularly for those who experience vision impairment. Smith [35] conducted a national study on the mobility problems of people with low vision as reported by clients and mobility practitioners. Results of this study indicated that lighting conditions and adaptation to lighting changes are the highest rated area of difficulty in mobility, with glare as the most frequently reported mobility problem [16]. Lighting enables the safe performance of mobility by illuminating different elements in the environment. Any factor that increases an individual's ability to detect objects in the environment will assist with safe mobility [23].

The function of an area determines the kind of lighting system that will be installed and whether the focus will be on task or ambient lighting [2]. Task lighting is using a luminaire that emits a strong bright beam in a relatively confined area to enable an individual to perform a specific activity, for example, a reading lamp or wayfinding light. In contrast ambient lighting is a wide diffuse beam that brightens the entire space, providing illumination for circulation and non-critical tasks; this is usually a traditional overhead ceiling light [7].

The primary function of a hallway is to enable safe traffic circulation. While other rooms use small pockets of task lighting to cater for more specific close work tasks, a hallway needs to provide a constant level of illumination [12], particularly as poorly lit areas in a hallway will create dangers such as object collision [7]. The illumination level of the hallway also plays an important role as it can assist the individual to adapt to a change in lighting conditions as they move from one level of lighting experienced in one room to another level of lighting in the next [12].

1.4. Level of illumination

Illumination is the term used to describe the amount of light arriving on a plane or a surface. It is measured in lumens per square metre (lux) [2]. The relationship between illumination level and visual performance has been described by Rea & Ouellette [34] as a "plateau followed by escarpment" effect. This statement describes how visual performance increases with an increase in illumination. This occurs up to a point where optimum visual performance is attained. The level of visual performance then remains constant even though illumination levels continue to increase (plateau). Eventually the illumination level is so high it begins to cause glare and visual performance declines (escarpment) [34]. Adequate illumination can be defined as the range of lux values at which the plateau occurs.

The importance of adequate illumination in travel situations was discussed by Long, Reiser and Hill [30]. They conducted a study investigating the variations in the indoor and outdoor loco-motor mobility of twenty two low vision adults. Their preliminary findings revealed that low illumination caused two to four times more mobility related incidents across travel environments [30].

More recent studies have demonstrated that low illumination causes reduced visual performance. In low illumination all subjects experienced a decrease in walking speed and an increase in mobility incidents involving object collision and veering off the pathway of travel [9, 13, 22, 26, 32].

Despite the amount of research conducted on illumination levels for mobility, there is quite a variation in the legislation for the lux level recommended in hallways as demonstrated in Table 1, with recommendations given by the Australian, United Kingdom and the United States lighting standards.

Table 1. Hallway illuminance recommendations

Location	**Illuminance recommendations (Lux)**
Australian Standards 4299 Adaptable Housing [37]	300
Australian Standards 1680.1 [38]	50
CIBSE (UK) - General [7]	100
CIBSE (UK) - for over the age of 65 [7]	225-300
IESNA Code (USA) -General [13]	50-75
IESNA Code (USA) - for over the age of 55 [13]	75-100

While the literature indicates that a high level of illumination is required to enable safe mobility no studies have been undertaken to determine a range of illumination levels that would enable the safe and independent mobility of people with vision impairment.

2. Research Questions

What range of lux values will provide an adequate level of illumination to enable an individual with vision impairment to safely and independently move through a residential hallway?

What type of lighting system is more effective at providing an adequate level of illumination: ambient lighting system, such as an overhead lighting system or a task lighting system such as a wayfinding light?

3. Method

A systematic review was conducted to synthesize the existing body of literature to determine what is currently known and unknown about illumination for people with vision impairment. It is anticipated that the results from this systematic literature review will aid in decision-making regarding the design of a residential lighting system.

The protocol that was employed to facilitate this systematic review process was supplied by the Home Modification and Maintenance Clearinghouse and is based on the Campbell Systematic Review Protocol and the Cochrane Systematic Review Protocol. It was selected because it is more inclusive of qualitative materials and provides a greater range of data relevant to home modifications [5].

3.1. Developing search terms

The HMM Systematic review protocol recommended refining the question into an operational format that would enable it to be researched systematically. This process could be undertaken by conducting a five part analysis of the research questions into, problem, intervention, outcome, comparison and target population based on Taylor's question refinement strategy [39].

Table 2. Question Refinement Strategy

Problem	Intervention	Outcome	Comparison	Target Population
Inadequate illumination	Wayfinding light system,	Safe and independent mobility	Overhead lighting	Vision Impairment

A list of search terms was then developed based on these five key components.

Table 3. List of search terms

Problem	Intervention	Outcome	Comparison	Target Population
Illumination	Floor	Mobility	Ceiling	Vision
Illuminance	Ground	Orientation	Above	Visual
Luminance	Lighting	Navigation	Overhead	Sight

Lumination	Wayfinding	Ambulation	Lighting	Impairment
Luminaire	LED	Travel		Impaired
Light	Phosphorescent	Locomotion		Disability
		Walk		Disabled
				Handicap
				Disorder

3.2. Search criteria

The strict inclusion and exclusion criteria described below were used to ensure that only articles of the utmost relevance were included as datum sources. These criteria were also used to determine the number of primary datum sources included in the study and were set to locate 20 to 50 articles that could be identified as suitable for analysis in the systematic review.

3.3. Inclusion Criteria

In order for material to be eligible for inclusion in this systematic review they had to correspond to all of the following criteria:

- All sources of literature must be attainable through the University of Sydney Library Network or via the World Wide Web Internet.
- All sources of literature must be written in English to eliminate the need for translation.
- All sources of literature must have been written within the last 50 year period. Most material printed prior to this time has been deemed to have little relevance as technology in home modifications and housing construction has changed considerably during this period [5].
- All sources of literature are relevant to the keywords; these keywords have been chosen carefully to take into account the differences in spelling, meaning and professional usage across all English speaking countries.
- All sources of literature must be based on studies that exclusively involve human subjects.
- During data extraction if the source of literature did not provide enough information under at least two of the subject headings on the matrix table, either person, environment or activity then it was rejected on the premise that it was not adequately informative to meet the needs of the review.
- Sources of literature from all levels of evidence were eligible for inclusion in the review, however, the limitation and potential bias in each was taken into account. The level of evidence hierarchy is described in Table 4. Each source of literature was weighed according to their level of evidence and potential for biasing the review.

3.4. Exclusion Criteria

If any of the material located during the data collection process met any of the following criteria they were automatically excluded from this systematic review:

- Written in a language other than English
- Written before 1954
- The study was conducted on non-human subjects
- Whole of subject textbooks because they tend to be of a very general nature and there is a high potential for bias in this material.
- Conference papers and editorials were excluded from the research because they are inaccessible to the University of Sydney Library Network.

3.5. Data searching

The data collection was conducted in accordance with the search strategy outlined in the HMM systematic review protocol. The protocol required the following literature sources to be thoroughly searched:

- The HMM Information Clearinghouse libraries existing collection of materials
- Standard electronic database search based on the Cochrane Systematic Review protocol guidelines
- World Wide Web search using the 'Google' and 'Google Scholar' search engine plus a search of identified potential websites
- Grey literature search
- Anecdotal evidence.
- Legislative and regulatory documents

Each literature source has its own search procedure that required various searching techniques, described in the following sections.

Using a search technique that encompassed all the various search terms enabled potential datum sources to be gathered. Each potential datum source was scanned for relevance and possible inclusion through a multi-stepped review process, illustrated in Figure 1.

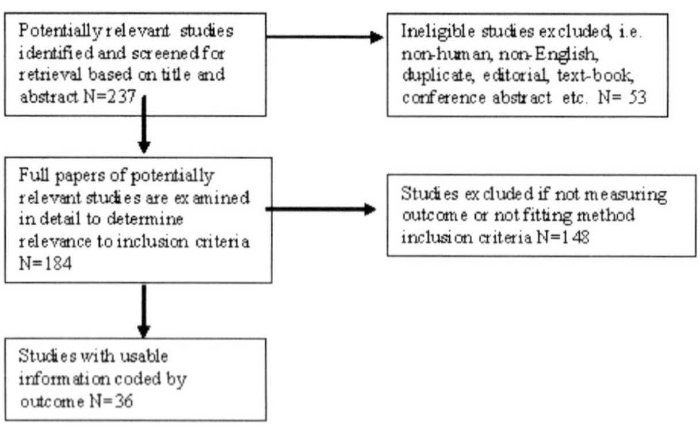

Figure 1: Flow chart of the review process [5].

The title and abstract was screened from each potential datum source. If this was deemed relevant a full text version of the study was obtained, read, summarized and evaluated against the data matrix to determine for a final time whether the source met the inclusion criteria and would be of benefit to the study.

4. Data analysis

We located 36 datum sources that met the inclusion criteria; these were assessed through a data matrix. This is a framework designed to code, appraise and systematically extract information from all the datum sources gathered in this study.

Sixteen legislative and regulatory documents were also included. Each document was reviewed and information of relevance was noted. A table was constructed to compare any similarities and differences among them.

5. Findings

Level of illumination was a feature of the environment that was of a great concern to a majority of the studies (72%) assessed in the data matrix. These studies investigated the performance of subjects who travelled through photopic and mesopic conditions. Their findings confirmed what was stated in the background review, that an increase in illumination will assist mobility performance [3, 13, 16, 17, 19, 25, 27, 28, 31, 40].

While these studies commented on illumination levels, few of them discussed the range of illumination levels that could be considered adequate. A number of the datum sources, particularly those obtained through the legislative and regulatory document search suggested illumination values that would satisfy the requirements of hallway lighting. There was a diverse range of values suggested by the datum sources and these started at 20 lux and extended up to 300 lux.

Hallways are used for a variety of activities and are not solely for the purpose of orientation and mobility. The illumination levels given in these regulatory documents took into consideration additional activities, such as checking clothing in the mirror, sorting the mail and buttoning a jacket. The aim of this study was to determine a range of lux values that will provide adequate illumination to enable safe and independent mobility. Therefore, it was important to consider studies that specifically analyzed the activity of mobility rather than those who assessed hallway lighting. Essentially there were two sets of studies that investigated the adequate level of illumination required for the activity of mobility; studies that investigated ambient lighting and those that analyzed task lighting, in particular wayfinding light systems.

Adequate illumination for a hallway to enable safe and independent mobility according to the datum sources can range between 20 lux to 40 lux. The Australian Standard 1680.0 – 1998 supplies the minimum electric lighting requirements to enable safe movement through a building. This standard states that a minimum illuminance of 20 lux should be provided throughout the space [38]. This value was supported in the study conducted by Watson [41] who discovered that 90% of subjects could perform the most difficult tasks at 20 lux [41]. The Australian Standard 1680.1 recommends a value of 40 lux as this value will be sufficient enough to enable the detection of task detail as well as navigating a safe pathway of travel through a crowded circulation space. From these studies it can be determined that adequate illumination for ambient hallway lighting to enable safe and independent mobility is within the range of 20 to 40 lux.

Whereas the studies above focused on ambient hallway lighting, other studies focused on emergency exit lighting, which can be considered a form of task lighting. Ambient lighting broadly lights the entire area allowing for a range of activities to be performed. Task lighting enables an individual to perform a specific activity; in the case of wayfinding lighting it is enabling the person to safely and independently move through the environment. The definition of adequate now has to satisfy the requirement that the level of illumination emitted from the wayfinding lighting system will enable safe mobility.

The most significant study concerned with the illumination level of wayfinding light systems was conducted by the Research Centre for Inclusive Environments. Their study analysed overhead and wayfinding lighting systems and analysed the illumination level each system supplied. They discovered that wayfinding systems with a low value of only 0.1 lux on the floor along the route was preferred to the conventional overhead system [44]. This was also confirmed in their later study that examined the effects of smoke on people's walking speed using overhead lighting and wayfinding provision [46]. Aizlewood and Weber [1] had similar findings, but discovered participants were able to safely move through the environment when wayfinding systems were as low as 0.05lux; however their subjects were fully sighted. These studies show that adequate illumination for wayfinding light systems to enable safe and independent mobility range from 0.05 to 1 lux.

6. Discussion

Lighting for orientation and mobility has been traditionally considered an activity that requires ambient lighting. This is because ambient lighting is capable of providing a wide diffuse beam that brightens the entire space, providing illumination for circulation and non-critical tasks [7].

The Royal Blind Society and the Centre for Lighting Research recommend increasing illumination to two or three times the recommended illumination levels in the legislative and regulatory documents [15]. This increase in illumination brightens the entire space, lighting all the features in the environment and enabling the performance of a number of activities [35].

Many studies have demonstrated that an increase in illumination can enable a safe performance of mobility with fewer mobility incidents and at a faster walking speed [4] [9, 10, 11, 24]. The level of illumination produced by wayfinding light systems is much lower (0.05 lux – 1 lux) than the recommended levels of illumination, yet subjects were able to move independently and safely with minimal mobility incidents and at a regular walking pace [1, 8, 41, 42, 43, 44].

One explanation for why safe mobility can be achieved at such a low level of illumination is because wayfinding light systems producing a task light are able to contrast with the environment emphasizing a safe pathway of travel. Ambient lighting illuminates the entire environment and for some people this can emphasize too many features in the environment causing visual confusion. The individual then has to navigate their own safe pathway of travel based on the physical layout of the environment and this is considerably more difficult than just following the illuminated pathway created by the wayfinding light system.

Another issue with ambient lighting is adapting to the high level of illumination required in the environment. The Royal Blind Society recommends 300 lux for hallway lighting to enable safe orientation and mobility [15]. For an individual transferring from a bright environment, very little dark light adaptation is required. An individual coming from a dark environment, for example going to the bathroom in the middle of the night and turning on the hallway light, has to suddenly adapt to the lighting conditions. For someone with vision impairment it will take from 2-6 minutes to adjust to these sudden changes in lighting conditions [6]. This is enough time for the individual to become disorientated and veer off the pathway of travel or collide with an object positioned in the hallway.

Wayfinding light systems can be considered a form of task lighting because they specifically illuminate the area required to enable the performance of safe mobility. This can be done effectively because the light system uses a low level of illumination that contrasts with the environment, emphasizing the pathway of travel. An ambient light system that increases the overall illumination of the environment. Home modification service providers should consider recommending an increase in contrast along the pathway of travel, by using a wayfinding light system, rather than recommending an overall increase in ambient illumination.

7. Conclusion

An adequate level of illumination for an ambient lighting system to enable safe movement through a building is 20 – 40 lux [37, 38, 41]. While adequate illumination for task lighting, such as wayfinding light systems can be 0.05 – 1 lux [1, 43, 46]

A major finding of this systematic review was the importance of contrast in the environment. This differs considerably to most of the research that was discussed in the background literature review. The focus of a considerable number of studies was on the illumination level required for people with vision impairment. The results of this systematic review concluded that a low level of illumination (0.05 – 1.0 lux) was sufficient for a lighting system to enable safe mobility, provided that the lighting system created a high contrast with the background environment

Acknowledgements

This material was produced from the work undertaken by Michala Pitch whilst on placement in the HMMinfo Clearinghouse. Michala's research thesis was supervised by Catherine Bridge and was originally published as an honours thesis. The project team gratefully acknowledges the financial and other support received from the NSW Department of Ageing, Disability and Home Care (DADHC) and the Commonwealth Home and Community Care Program without which this work would not have been possible.

The authors would also like to acknowledge the contribution of many experts from the Royal Blind Society, Guide Dogs Association and the lighting research industry who generously gave their time. Without them all sharing their ideas, perspectives and information this knowledge could not have been generated.

References

[1] Aizlewood, C. E., & Webber, G. M. B. (1995). Escape route lighting: Comparison of human performance with traditional lighting and wayfinding systems. *Lighting Research and Technology, 27*(3), 133-143.

[2] Bean, R. (2004). *Lighting - interior and exterior*. Oxford: Architectural Press.

[3] Black, A., Lovie-Kitchin, J. E., Woods, R. L., Arnold, N., Byrnes, J., & Murrish, J. (1997). Mobility performance with Retinitis Pigamentosa. *Clinical and Experimental Optometry, 80*(1).

[4] Boyce, P. R., & Sanford, L. J. (2000). Lighting to enhance visual capabilities. In B. Silverstone, M. A. Lang, B. P. Rosenthal & E. E. Faye (Eds.), *The lighthouse handbook on vision impairment and vision rehabilitation* (Vol. Vol 1: vision impairment, pp. 617-636). New York: Oxford University Press.

[5] Bridge, C., & Phibbs, P. (2003). *Protocol Guidelines for systematic reviews of home modification information to inform best practice.* Sydney: Home maintenance and modification clearing house, the University of Sydney.

[6] Carter, K. (1989). Assessment of lighting. In R. T. Jose (Ed.), *Understanding Low Vision* (pp. 403-414). New York: American Foundation for the Blind.

[7] Chartered Institution of Building Services Engineers. (1997). *Lighting for communal residential buildings, Lighting Guide LG9:1997.* London: Chartered Institution of Building Services Engineers.

[8] Cook, G. K., Wright, M. S., Webber, G. M. B., & Bright, K. T. (1999). Emergency lighting and wayfinding provision systems for visually impaired people: Phase II of a study. *Lighting Research and Technology, 31*(2), 43-49.

[9] Cornelissen, W., Bootsma, A., & Kooijman, A. C. (1995). Object perception by visually impaired people at different light levels. *Vision research, 35*(1), 161-168.

[10] Cornelissen, W., Kooijman, A. C., Bootsma, A., & Van der Wildt, G. J. (1994). Light and objects; perceiving 'the real thing'. In A. C. Kooijman, P. L. Looijestijn, J. A. Welling & G. J. Van der Wildt (Eds.), *Low vision - Research and new developments in rehabilitation* (pp. 78-84). Amsterdam: IOS press.

[11] Cornelissen, W. F., Kooijman, A. C., Van Schoot, E. A. J., Bootsma, A., & Van der Wildt, G. (1994). Optimizing illumination for visually impaired persons: comparing subjective and objective criteria. In A. C. Kooijman, P. L. Looijestijn, J. A. Welling & G. J. Van der Wildt (Eds.), *Low vision* (pp. 68-77). Amsterdam: IOS press.

[12] De Chiara, J., Panero, J., & Zelnik, M. (1991). *Time saver standards for interior design and space planning* (2nd ed.). New York: McGraw Hill.

[13] Dickinson, C. (1998). *Low vision - principles and practice*. Oxford: Butterworth Heinemann.

[14] Elliott, D. B., Bullimore, M. A., Patla, A. E., & Whitaker, D. (1996). Effect of a cataract simulation on clinical and real world vision. *British Journal of Opthamology, 80*(9), 799-804.

[15] Ferronato, L., Gialouris, C., & Phillips, L. (2002, 19-20 September, 2002). *Seeing the light: the importance of illumination for low vision and the older population.* Paper presented at the OT Australia NSW Conference, Sydney, Australia.

[16] Geruschat, D. R., & Smith, A. J. (1997). Low vision and mobility. In B. B. Blasch, W. R. Wiener & R. L. Welsh (Eds.), *Foundations of orientation and mobility* (2nd ed., pp. 60-80). New York: AFB press.

[17] Geruschat, D. R., & Turano, K. A. (2002). Connecting research on Retinitis Pigamentosa to the Practice of Orientation and Mobility. *Journal of visual impairment and blindness, February*, 69-83.

[18] Golledge, R. G. (1991). Tactual strip maps as navigational aids. *Journal of Visual Impairment & Blindness*, 296-301.

[19] Hassan, S. E., Lovie-Kitchin, J. E., Woods, R. L., & Soong, G. P.-Y. (2000). Orientation and mobility in age-related macular degeneration. *Visual Impairment Research, 1*(3), 175-180.

[20] Jacobsen, R. D. (1998). Cognitive mapping without sight: four preliminary studies of spatial learning. *Journal of Environmental Psychology, 18*, 289-305.

[21] Jansson, G. (1991). The control of locomotion when vision is reduced or missing. In A. E. Patla (Ed.), *Adaptability of human gait* (pp. 333-357). North-Holland: Elsevier Science Publishers.

[22] Julian, W. G. (1983). The design of the visual environment of the aged partially sighted. *Architectural Science Review, 26*(3/4), 112-115.

[23] Kaufman, J. E., & Haynes, H. (1981). *IES lighting handbook.* North America: Illuminated Engineering Society of North America.

[24] Kuyk, T., & Elliott, J. L. (1999). Visual factors and mobility in persons with age-related macular degeneration. *Journal of Rehabilitation Research, 36*(4), 303-311.

[25] Kuyk, T., & Elliott, J. L. (1999). Visual factors and mobility in persons with age-related macular degeneration. *Journal of Rehabilitation Research and Development, 36*(4), 303-313.

[26] Kuyk, T., Elliott, J. L., & Fuhr, P. S. W. (1998). Visual correlates of mobility in real world settings in older adults with low vision. *Optometry and vision sciences, 75*(7), 538-547.

[27] Kuyk, T., Elliott, J. L., & Patti, S. W. (1998a). Visual correlates of mobility in real world settings in older adults with low vision. *Optometry and vision science, 75*(7), 538-547.

[28] Kuyk, T., Elliott, J. L., & Patti, S. W. (1998b). Visual correlates of obstacle avoidance in adults with low vision. *Optometry and vision science, 75*(3), 174-182.

[29] Long, R. G., Boyette, L. W., & Griffin-Shirley, N. (1996). Older persons and community travel: the effect of visual impairment. *Journal of Visual Impairment & Blindness*, 302-313.

[30] Long, R. G., Reiser, J. J., & Hill, E. W. (1990). Mobility in individuals with moderate visual impairment. *Journal of Visual Impairment & Blindness, 84*(2), 111-118.

[31] Long, R. G., Rieser, J. J., & Hill, E. W. (1990). Mobility in individuals with moderate visual impairment. *Journal of Rehabilitation Research, 84*(3), 111-118.

[32] Lovie-Kitchin, J., Woods, R. L., & Black, A. (1997). *Effect of illuminance on the mobility performance of adults with retinitis pigmentosa*. Retrieved 21/06/04, 2004

[33] Patla, A. E. (1991). Visual control of human locomotion. In A. E. Patla (Ed.), *Adaptability of human gait; implications for the control of locomotion* (Vol. 78, pp. 55-97). North Holland: Elsevier Science Publishers.

[34] Rea, M. S., & Ouelette, M. J. (1998). Visual Performance using reaction times. *Lighting Research and Technology, 20*(4), 139-153.

[35] Smith, F. K., & Bertolone, F. J. (1986). *Bringing interiors to light: the principles and practices of lighting design*. New York: Whitney Library of Design.

[36] Soong, G., & Lovie-Kitchin, J. (2001). Does mobility performance of visually impaired adults improve immediately after orientation and mobility training. *Optometry and vision sciences, 78*(9), 657-666.

[37] Standards Australia. (1990). *1680.1 - 1990 Interior Lighting*. Australia: Building code of Australia.

Standards Australia. (1995). *AS 4299 - 1995 Adaptable Housing*. Homebush: Standards Association of Australia.

[38] Standards Australia. (1998). *1680.0 - 1998 Interior Lighting Part 0: Safe Movement* (Vol. 1680.0). Homebush: Standards Australia.

[39] Taylor, C. (2000). *Evidence based practice for occupational therapists*. Oxford: Blackwell Science.

[40] Turano, K. A., Broman, A. T., Bandeen-Roche, K., Munoz, B., Rubin, G. S., & West, S. K. (2004). Association of visual field loss and mobility performance in older adults: Salisbury Eye Evaluation Study. *Optometry and vision science, 81*(5), 298-307.

[41] Watson, G. C. (2002). *Emergency evacuation in aged care establishments with a particular emphasis on illumination.*Unpublished manuscript, Sydney.

[42] Webber, G. M. B., Hallman, P. J., & Salvidge, A. C. (1988). Movement under emergency lighting: comparison between standard provisions and photoluminescent markings. *Lighting Research and Technology, 20*(4), 167-175.

[43] Wright, M., Bright, K., & Cook, G. (1996). *Escape route lighting for people with vision impairment*. Retrieved 12th July, 2005, from www.rics-foundation.org/publish/download.aspx?did=2427

[44] Wright, M., Cook, G., & Bright, K. (1997). Design Guidance for emergency escape route lighting. *Access by design*(73).

[45] Wright, M. S., Cook, G. K., & Webber, G. M. B. (1999). Emergency lighting and wayfinding provision systems for visually impaired people: Phase 1 of a study. *Lighting Research and Technology, 31*(2), 35-42.

[46] Wright, M. S., Cook, G. K., & Webber, G. M. B. (2002). *The effects of smoke on people's walking speeds using overhead lighting and wayguidance provision*. Retrieved 11th July, 2005, from http://www.rdg.ac.uk/ie/research/eewp/bstnspeedfin.pdf

[47] Yablonski, M. S. (2000). Functional orientation and mobility. In B. Silverstone, M. A. Lang, B. P. Rosenthal & E. E. Faye (Eds.), *The lighthouse handbook on vision and vision rehabilitation* (Vol. 2, pp. 855-867). New York: Oxford university press.

Promoting Independence for Older Persons with Disabilities
W.C. Mann and A. Helal (Eds.)
IOS Press, 2006

Universal Design in Aging in Place Senior Housing: A Pilot Study of Resident's Perspectives

Duncan PARK[a, 1]
Department of Occupational Therapy, School of Health Professions, University of Missouri – Columbia, Columbia MO USA

Abstract. Universal design can allow people to age in place. The purpose of this research is to assess the safety, accessibility, functionality, and aesthetic appeal of universal design in a state of Missouri pilot project for senior residential living. Resident rating was higher for universal design features than for non-universal design in all four categories.

Keywords. Universal design, home modifications, functional barriers

Introduction

A recent survey of 2,000 Americans over age 45 revealed that more than 80% want to live in one residence as long as possible, and this response increased to over 90% for those over 65 [1]. Two-thirds of the respondents indicated they would like to see more homes built with features that allow people to remain in them as they age. However, with age, disability often limits functional activity in conventional homes. Half of older people report one or more disabilities, and one-third describes their disability as severe [2]. Yet, disability is increasingly seen as environmental rather than personal [3]. Christenson [4] quotes Margaret Wylde, a universal design proponent, who estimates "that at one time or another, 90% of us will be 'disabled' by conventional building design".

Universal design seeks to eliminate these barriers. Supporting this objective, current occupational therapy literature describes home modification as optimizing human performance by creating environments that are physically accessible, functional, and safe [5]. North Carolina State University's Center for Universal Design has compiled a detailed array of features that integrate these three components into lived spaces [6].

Aesthetic considerations figure prominently when people create or modify home environments and this is also reflected in occupational therapy literature. Universal design has been described as comfortable, emotionally accessible, good-looking, and especially "invisible" [3, 4]. The unobtrusiveness of these environments is not just a matter of seamless integration, but implies a concerted effort to avoid stigmatizing users. By creating spaces with broad aesthetic appeal, universal design seeks to eliminate what Falta [7] calls "the us-and-them syndrome".

1. Background

Few studies have assessed the effects of environmental modifications [8]. Researchers who have examined specialized living environments often study "accessible housing" or features that respond to specific medical diagnoses, but do not include design that accommodates all people [9, 10].

Crist [11] compared reports of older adults on the quality of life experienced in various types of dwellings, including collective housing. The author found that among the quality of life indicators relevant to housing were access to resources, and responsiveness of the environment to personal needs. The research found that current satisfaction was highest among personal home dwellers, while those living in specialized housing reported the greatest overall satisfaction. The author concluded that "good 'person-environment match' will maximize individual quality of life" [11]. Assessing the effect of universal design features was not part of the scope of this study. However, the results demonstrate the need to investigate how features of a home, in particular those intended to optimize functioning across the lifespan, affect resident satisfaction.

The impact of universal design on accessibility and functionality was explicitly evaluated in multifamily housing units in Montreal, Quebec [7]. This was done using a post-occupancy evaluation (POE), a method that assesses the effect of the built environment on a resident's functional needs. The objective of Falta's [7] study was to assess the reaction of persons both with and without disabilities who already lived in these units in order to determine the validity of universal design principles for a wide population range. Implementing the POE involved development of a questionnaire that measured the degree of satisfaction with the housing unit design, focusing specifically on access and function. Determining user reaction to the aesthetic quality of the units was not among the research objectives. Nevertheless, many subjects expressed lack of awareness that universal design principles had been integrated into the buildings, while others expressed dissatisfaction with the comfort and attractiveness of some elements. Despite mixed feedback on aesthetics, the results of the study convinced the author that the overall functional needs of persons with and without specific limitations were met by the "universal access" housing units.

In addition to post-occupancy evaluations, other tools have been devised for evaluating the effectiveness of lived environments in assuring the safety, accessibility and optimal function of residents. However, the purpose of many of these tools is to adapt environments to specific individuals, the very antithesis of universal design which favors inclusion of all people [6, 8, 12].

To establish a solid body of evidence for the effectiveness of universal home design, the call is going out for therapists to collect anthropomorphic data [13]. Other researchers advocate a shift toward more qualitative methods to achieve this goal [7]. Ringaert [10] proposes the development of a new environmental assessment tool based on universal design principles, eliciting feedback from residents by means of questionnaires and interviews, and tracking results. Trachtman et al. [3] also encourage input from those living in universal design environments and the study of spaces that incorporate this design ethic. Failure to explore the effects of universal design on consumers will create "serious barriers to the shift from concept to practice" [13].

2. Purpose of Study

The purpose of this research was to examine the effectiveness of universal design homes in providing safe, accessible, functional and aesthetically-pleasing environments as perceived by senior residents of an aging-in-place living community. A better understanding of the lived experience of this population will help occupational therapists make evidence-based recommendations for environmental modifications.

3. Method

Research was conducted at a prototypical aging-in-place senior living community where residents share public spaces and have individual apartments of various configurations. Open less than a year at the time of the study, the design of the building and grounds was a collaborative effort of various medical, environmental design, and health professionals, including occupational therapists. The expressed goal was to provide an environment that would help seniors maintain independence [14]. The present study used structured interviews based on a 65-item questionnaire for data collection.

3.1. Participants

Recruitment took place at two informational meetings in public areas of the facility. All residents were invited to attend through posted announcements and flyers. It was emphasized to those present at the meetings that participation in the study was voluntary and the individual responses of anyone choosing to participate would remain confidential. The following were exclusion criteria: living less than one month at the residence, physical or cognitive deficits impacting successful understanding and completion of the questionnaire, and belonging to a vulnerable population as judged by an affiliated nursing care agency. A convenience sample of nineteen consenting and eligible participants was gathered ($n=19$).

3.2. Instrument

The questionnaire had two components: Demographic information and rating of environmental features of the residence.

Demographic Information. Each questionnaire contained eight items that identified each participant's age group, gender, former housing type, date of arrival at the aging-in-place residence, current apartment configuration (studio, one-bedroom, etc.), ambulation status, driving status, and adaptations made to individual apartments since arrival.

Perspectives on environmental features of the residence. The fifty-seven items in this section of the questionnaire were adapted from guidelines published by the Center for Universal Design at North Carolina State University [6]. Table 1 shows some sample questions.

These items were organized by headings identifying the area of the residential environment: Entrances and walkways, public spaces, and individual apartments (including kitchen and bath sections). Under each heading in random

Table 1. Sample Questions by Heading

Entrances and Walkways	**Poor**	**Fair**	**Average**	**Very Good**	**Excellent**
Safety of entrances and walkways in wet and icy weather?	1	2	3	4	5
Public Spaces	**Poor**	**Fair**	**Average**	**Very Good**	**Excellent**
Ease of passing in hallways?	1	2	3	4	5
Individual Residences	**Poor**	**Fair**	**Average**	**Very Good**	**Excellent**
Attractiveness of the main living area?	1	2	3	4	5

order, questions rated resident perspective in one of four categories: safety, functionality, accessibility, or aesthetics. A Likert-type scale from 1 (poor) to 5 (excellent) was used to measure these independent variables. Four items were subsequently judged as inadmissible and eliminated due to absence of the feature or lack of resident experience in its use.

3.3. Procedure

The University of Missouri Health Sciences Institutional Review Board granted an expedited review and approved the research procedures. The residence administration also gave formal permission for the study.

Evaluation of Residence Building. Using the same guidelines for universal design incorporated into the resident questionnaire, the researcher made a detailed evaluation of the interior and exterior public areas. Two unoccupied individual apartments were also evaluated, an "alcove" or L-shaped space with contiguous living and sleeping areas, and a one-bedroom unit with these areas separated by a door. The two-bedroom apartments were tenant-occupied at the time of study but observation verified comparable features. All these apartment types had a kitchen, bath, walk-in closet, laundry area, and outdoor patio. Features of the residential environment corresponding to questionnaire items were then judged as either compliant or non-compliant with universal design guidelines.

Interviews. To enhance participation and accurate completion of the questionnaire, participants scheduled one-on-one interviews. Informed consent was obtained. Individual interviews were conducted by the same interviewer over a ten-day period.

3.4. Data Analysis

Quantitative data from this study was summarized from questionnaire responses using descriptive statistics. Outcomes of the compiled data are in the form of aggregate figures, percentages, means (*M*) and standard deviations (*SD*) (See Appendix A). The items from the questionnaire targeting the four specific areas of the research question (safety, functionality, accessibility, aesthetics) were combined to form mean averages.

4. Results

Demographic results are detailed in Table 2. The majority of study participants (95%) were aged 70 – 89 years. Both males (37%) and females (63%) were represented. A majority were driving and ambulating without the use of assistive devices. Over two-thirds of residents had come to this senior housing community from their own single-family dwellings, and nearly equal numbers of residents currently lived in one-bedroom (42%) and two-bedroom (47%) apartments. The only open-ended question in the study instrument asked residents to identify any changes that had been made to their individual apartment since arrival.

Sixty-three percent reported some kind of modification. These ranged from minor changes (the addition of doors to the closet entrance, a medicine cabinet

Table 2. Findings Related to Resident Demographics (*n=19*)

Age group		
	60-69:	0%
	70-79:	37%
	80-89:	58%
	90-	5%
Gender	Male:	37%
	Female:	63%
Driving status	Drive:	68%
	Don't drive:	32%
Changes made to apartment:		
	Yes:	63%
	No:	37%
Former housing		
	Care facility:	11%
	Condo:	21%
	House:	68%
	Apartment:	0%
Type of apartment		
	Two-bedroom:	47%
	One-bedroom:	42%
	Alcove:	11%
	Studio:	0%
Ambulation		
	Without aid:	68%
	With aid:	32%

(One participant used wheelchair outdoors)

above the bathroom counter or a grab bar outside the shower area) to major changes (the conversion of a garage or adjacent one bedroom apartment into additional living space). Changes to apartments were evaluated for possible confounding of independent variables. However, in each case, evaluation of the modified feature harmonized with the design of existing features in the same heading and category.

The building evaluation revealed that of the 53 items studied, 35 related to universal design and 18 to non-universal design features (See Table 3). Two-thirds (66%) of the residential environments studied, therefore, incorporated universal design principles, while one-third (34%) did not.

Table 3. Number of Survey Questions by Category and by Design Type Following Evaluation of Residence Building

Category	Universal Design Features	Non-Universal Design Features	
Safety	8	2	
Functionality	9	7	
Accessibility	6	4	
Aesthetics	12	4	
Total	**35**	**18**	**53**
(Questions Eliminated: 4)			

A key finding of the study is the relationship that appears when resident ratings of design features are compared. Universal design features were rated from approximately ½ point to more than one point higher than non-universal design in all categories surveyed. This outcome appears to confirm the researcher's hypothesis that building aging-in-place senior housing according to universal design guidelines would have a positive life impact from the resident's perspective. Tables 4a & 4b illustrate this relationship.

Table 4a. Comparison of Universal with Non-Universal Design Features in Categories of Safety, Functionality, Accessibility, and Aesthetics

Category	Universal Design	Non-Universal Design
Safety	**4.17**	**3.08**
Functionality	**4.24**	**3.69**
Accessibility	**4.25**	**3.59**
Aesthetics	**4.32**	**3.76**
Overall	**4.25**	**3.62**

Table 4b. Chart of Categories Rated

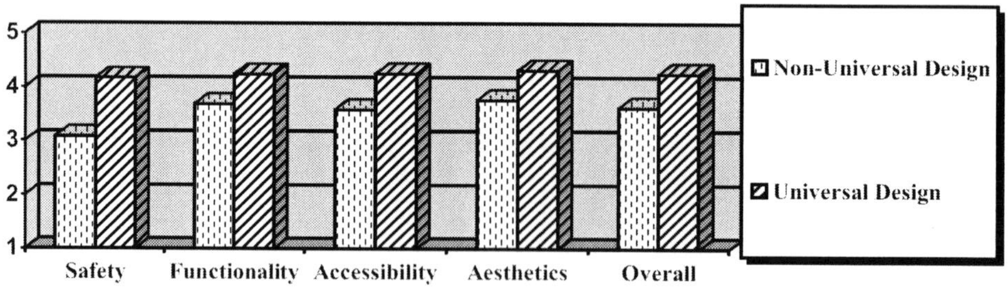

The questionnaire also identifies particular areas that the residents perceive as especially supportive and others that are highly challenging. Visibility of someone approaching the apartment from an outside door, access onto patio areas, and attractiveness of the public areas were the most highly rated items, almost invariably receiving responses of "very good" and "excellent". Other features of the residence building were viewed less favorably. The three most challenging aspects of the environment to residents all centered on the individual kitchen area: ability of the kitchen to accommodate more than one person at a time, reaching items in kitchen cabinets, and maneuvering large items from kitchen shelves.

The three features identified by residents as most supportive reflected universal design principles, whereas the three features perceived as most challenging were non-universal in design.

Mean averages show that residents of this aging-in-place living community perceive their home as well above average in functionality, accessibility, and aesthetic appeal. The safety of both universal design and non-universal design features, while still rated above average, received lower marks than any of the other categories.

The questionnaire was formatted to assess the environment from the exterior to the interior and from public to personal spaces. One interesting result of this construction was the opportunity it afforded to observe the progression of universal design implementation through the building. Every feature of the public spaces assessed during the building evaluation conformed to universal design standards. Evaluation of personal spaces reveals that universal design was reflected in less than half (17 of 35) of the apartment features measured. Table 5 graphically represents the resident's comparative levels of satisfaction. Analysis of these results shows residents find their private apartments somewhat less responsive to their needs than the public spaces.

Table 5. Public and Personal Spaces: Incorporation of Universal Design and the Resident's Perspective.

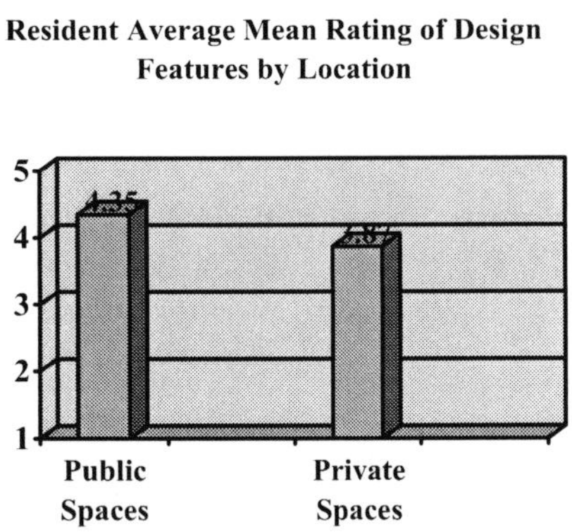

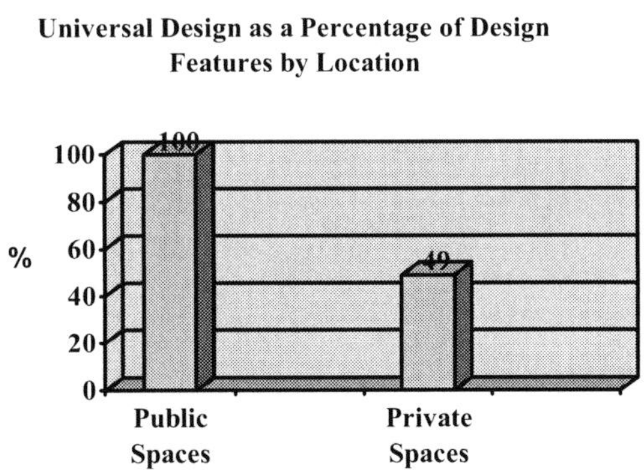

Discussion

The present study concluded that the majority of design elements in the residential environment surveyed are universal, enabling maximum participation by all users yet remaining virtually "invisible".

Results of this study provide preliminary evidence that the universal design approach to environmental modification is inclusive of older adults and elicits a positive response from resident users. The ability of universal design to provide a functional, accessible, safe and attractive home to individuals who wish to age in place was demonstrated.

Although aesthetic considerations appear in rehabilitation literature, a health professions database search reveals study of this construct generally has been limited to medical settings rather than personal environments. The findings of this study indicate a relationship between the perception of comfort and attractiveness of a home (aesthetics) and its ability to promote productive activity, mobility, and safety. Although care should be taken not to infer cause and effect from these comparisons, further study may reveal correlations between the presence of universal design features in the built environment and the type and quality of resident response.

While cost, amenities, autonomy, and other factors influence the type of housing seniors choose, aging-in-place facilities may have particular appeal to those in robust health. The demographic data of this study show that a significant majority of residents have relatively little functional impairment as measured by reports of independent walking and driving, in spite of the fact that all those surveyed were age 70 or older. The overall positive reaction to nearly all elements of the residence facility, therefore, may be partly due to the fact that seniors who move there are not experiencing the limitations that universal design accommodates.

One explanation for the large percentage of residents reporting changes to their apartments may be the limited number of universal design features built into these spaces. Kitchens, in particular, present challenges to older adults, including reach, grasp, bending, lifting, mobility and safety. This is confirmed by the collective perceptions of this study's participants. Kane [15] observes that kitchens designed to be supportive of all age groups improve functional activity.

It would be helpful to conduct a longitudinal study of the variables examined here to see whether the gap in satisfaction between universal design and traditional design features of the building will widen over time. Although this might be predicted on the basis of the holistic underpinnings of universal design, it is possible both design types would register declines in favorable response as is already the case in the area of safety relative to other aspects of user satisfaction.

5. Limitations

The instrument developed by the researcher of this study serves as an initial effort to create an assessment tool for universal design environments. The nearly limitless configurations of built environments and the range of human abilities and health status make such an undertaking vastly challenging. Therefore, the assessment of available model apartments as performed in this study seems inadequate to fully represent the lived experience of resident users.

A further limitation is difficulty in assessing the aesthetic construct. The response of residents to the aesthetic aspects of universal design may have overlapped considerably with unrelated design features, particularly the finishes, furnishings, and design style of the public spaces.

Self-selection and the limited sample size available for this study restrict the application of the findings to broad populations. Future research could encompass all aging-in-place pilot programs in a state or compare other housing types that integrate universal design.

6. Implications for the Future

Aging-in-place is a relatively new concept in housing design and healthcare service delivery and one that fits well with both the universal design approach and occupational therapy's view that a person's surroundings can enhance independence in valued life activities. As demand for this type of housing grows, public and private agencies are attempting to place it in the long-term care continuum [14]. This study and further research can contribute to the direction aging-in-place senior housing will take.

Understanding the reaction of people living in one such residential community gives insight into how successfully their surroundings will age with them. The study provides a snapshot of a particular moment in time and the current perception of need expressed by residents. While the response to universal design in this study was modest, a trend of support for it is beginning to appear. Only time and additional investigation will tell if this trend will establish universal design as a significant contributor to the success of aging-in-place senior housing.

Clearly, it is in the best interests of architects, builders, and healthcare professionals to understand the evolution of the functional needs of their clients across the life spectrum. Joe [16] quotes Morris, as saying, "we need to sensitize OT practitioners on the one hand and architects and designers on the other on how they can best work together – as well as with users – to create universal design products and help individuals make wise choices". It is far better from both the standpoint of human health and cost-effective delivery of services to incorporate evidence-based design solutions from the start of the building process, rather than alter the structure of a space and retrofit adaptive features as the resident undergoes continual life changes [10].

7. Conclusions

If the findings of this research are enlarged upon by additional studies with greater sample sizes and application of correlational analysis, universal design may be confirmed as an aesthetically-pleasing alternative to traditional design that promotes function, mobility, and safety through the lifespan. In that case, occupational therapists will no doubt continue to embrace it as an adjunct to a holistic view of wellness that includes the role of environment in occupational performance.

On the other hand, research may reveal universal design to be limited in meeting the infinite array of user needs and wants by its very all-inclusive nature. Occupational therapy is well-suited to developing environments tailored to promoting optimum health, social participation, and personal achievement, picking up where universal design leaves off. In either case, it is hoped that in time occupational therapy will become less focused on persuading people of the need for better environments, and more centered on assisting people to create the environments they need in order to age in place [3].

Acknowledgements

The author thanks the faculty of the Department of Occupational Therapy, University of Missouri, Columbia, particularly Department Chair Dr. Guy L. McCormack, Ph.D., OTR/L, FAOTA and Clinical Instructor, Sherry Borcherding, OTR/L who assisted in refining the study and the participants of the study who offered their valuable time and insights.

References

[1] AARP (2000). *Fixing to stay: A national survey on housing and home modification issues.* Washington, DC: Author.

[2] Administration on Aging, U.S. Department of Health and Human Services. (2003). *A profile of older Americans: 2003.* Retrieved October 11, 2004, from http://research.aarp.org/general/profile_2003.pdf

[3] Trachtman, L.H., Mace, R.L., Young, L.C., & Pace, R.J. (1999). The universal design home: Are we ready for it? *Physical and Occupational Therapy in Geriatrics, 16* (3/4), 1-18.

[4] Christenson, M.A. (1999). Embracing universal design [Electronic version]. *OT Practice, 4* (9), 12-15, 25.

[5] Cumming, R.G., Thomas, M., Szonyi, G., Frampton, G., Salkeld, G., & Clemson, L. (2001). Adherence to occupational therapist recommendations for home modifications for falls prevention. *American Journal of Occupational Therapy, 55*, 641-648.

[6] Universal design in housing. (2003). Retrieved September 27, 2004, from North Carolina State University, Center for Universal Design web site: http://www.design.ncsu.edu/cud/pdf_files/UDinHousing.doc

[7] Falta, P.L. (1999). Postoccupancy evaluation of universally accessible multifamily housing units. In E. Steinfeld & G. S. Danford (Eds.), Enabling environments: Measuring the impact of environment on disability and rehabilitation. (pp. 351-371). New York: Kluwer Academic.

[8] Christenson, M., Sabata, D., Fagan, L.A., Shamberg, S., & Carter, M.A. (2004). Report on environmental intervention as an area for specialty certification. American Occupational Therapy Association. Retrieved September 23, 2004, from http://www.aota.org/members/area16/docs/env.pdf

[9] Gitlin LN., Schinfeld S., Winter L., Corcoran M,. Boyce AA., & Hauck W. (2002). Evaluating home environments of persons with dementia: Interrater reliability and validity of the Home Environmental Assessment Protocol (HEAP). *Disability and Rehabilitation. 24*(1/3), 59-71.

[10] Ringaert, L., (2003). Universal design of the built environment to enable occupational performance. In L. Letts, P. Rigby, & D. Stewart (Eds.), *Using environments to enable occupational performance* (pp. 97-116). Thorofare, NJ: Slack.

[11] Christ, A.C., (1999). Does quality of life vary with different types of housing among older persons? A pilot study. *Physical & Occupational Therapy in Geriatrics, 16*, (3/4), 101-116.

[12] Pynoos, J. & Nishita, C.M., (2003). The Cost and Financing of Home Modifications in the United States. *Journal of Disability Policy Studies, 14* (2), 68-73.

[13] Connell, B.R. & Sanford, J.A. (1999). Research implications of universal design. In E. Steinfeld & G. S. Danford (Eds.), Enabling environments: Measuring the impact of environment on disability and rehabilitation. (pp. 35-57). New York: Kluwer Academic.

[14] Marek, K.D., & Rantz, M.J. (2000). Aging in place: A new model for long term care. *Nursing Administration Quarterly, 24* (3), 1-11.

[15] Kane, R.A. (2001). Long-term care and a good quality of life: Bringing them closer together. *The Gerontologist, 41,* 293-304.

[16] Joe, B.E., (1998). Where OT and architecture come together. *OT Week, 12* (1), 16, 19.

Chapter 4

Assistive Devices

W.C. Mann and A. Helal (Eds.)
IOS Press, 2006

Effective and Confidential Communication of Prescription Information: Accommodating the Blind and Visually-Impaired

John LITTLE[a,1]
Healthcare law private practice.

Abstract. Individuals with vision disabilities face unique difficulties in their attempt to utilize prescription information such as medication descriptions, dosage instructions, side-effect warnings and other information often considered to be detailed and complex, yet essential. Similarities in container shapes and sizes along with having multiple prescription medications compound these problems. Sighted pharmacy customers are obvious beneficiaries of U.S. state and federal requirements obligating pharmacies to provide detailed, written medication information to prescription containers. These requirements govern both the content of the information and the duty to physically affix or attach the content to prescription containers. The U.S. Americans with Disabilities Act (ADA) addresses the obligation of pharmacies to provide their blind and visually-impaired customers with effective auxiliary communication aids. The U.S. Health Insurance Portability and Accountability Act (HIPAA) privacy regulations require pharmacies to permit their customers, individually, to request that communications of the customer's protected health information be made by alternative means. Currently, the most commonly utilized auxiliary method of communicating prescription medication information to the blind and visually-impaired is face-to-face counseling. This method is also one of the most ineffective at communicating complex, detailed medication information to this population and can be considered one of the most burdensome methods that may be implemented by pharmacies. Recent technological advances, however, have led to the development of Audible Prescription Labeling Systems (APLS) specifically designed for blind and visually-impaired pharmacy customers, providing such customers, for the first time, a meaningful opportunity to enjoy the ability to keep their prescription medication information private. While each of the available APLS communication aids has a relatively insignificant impact on pharmacy expenses and operations, they do vary in communication effectiveness. One of the four available APLS communication aids on the market overcomes issues related to communication effectiveness and pharmacy burden by utilizing text-to-speech technology and a Radio Frequency Identification (RFID) enabled label that securely affixes to any type of prescription medication container, including odd-shaped glass and plastic bottles, blister packs and boxes.

Introduction

Blind and visually-impaired pharmacy customers face unique difficulties in their attempt to utilize prescription information such as medication descriptions, dosage instructions, side-effect warnings and other information often considered to be detailed and complex, yet essential. These customers' difficulties are compounded dramatically by simple issues such as similarities in container shapes and sizes and having been prescribed more than one medication. While sighted pharmacy customers are obvious beneficiaries of state and federal requirements that detailed written information accompany prescription medications, the blind and visually-impaired require special accommodation in order to benefit from such information. Absent the provision of effective auxiliary communication aids, blind and visually-impaired pharmacy customers are incapable of taking advantage of the same goods, services and privileges available to sighted customers.

However, federal laws do exist which address the obligation of pharmacies to provide their blind and visually-impaired customers with effective auxiliary communication aids. Until recently, provision of the only such aids available has been viewed either as ineffective or as creating an undue burden on business operations. Fortunately, technological advances over the past few years, including Audible Prescription Labeling Systems (APLS) utilizing Radio Frequency Identification (RFID), now allow pharmacies to offer truly effective auxiliary communication aids to the blind and visually-impaired efficiently and economically, with only minor, insignificant alterations to their current operations.

1. Mandatory Prescription Medication Label Information

The nature and extent of medication information that pharmacies are required to provide their customers has been the subject of complex, overlapping and evolving state and federal regulation. The justification for this regulation is readily apparent upon review of recent reports estimating the number of deaths and other adverse health consequences related to medication errors in the United States each year.[1],[2],[3] The Food and Drug Administration's Center for Drug Evaluation and Research states that "medication errors cause at least one death every day and injure approximately 1.3 million people annually in the United States."[4] The problem is so significant that the American Pharmacists Association stresses that prescription medication users should "double check the label and the contents" prior to taking a medication.[5] The association also warns prescription users to "read the label and follow the directions. Medications are powerful, that's why they work. But they can cause harm as well, particularly if they are not used correctly. Follow the directions on the label."[5] Recognizing the importance of the availability of accurate and complete medication information, federal law establishes severe penalties related to the delivery of false, misleading or incomplete information attached to or included with prescription medications.

1.1. Content Requirements

The federal Food, Drug, and Cosmetic Act (FDCA) includes in the definition of "misbranding" any written, printed or graphic matter on or accompanying a drug which is false or misleading in any particular.[6] Section 201(n) of the FDCA describes the concept of misleading and specifically provides that in determining whether the labeling of a drug is misleading, "there shall be taken into account (among other things) not only representations made ... but also the extent to which the labeling or advertising fails to reveal facts material ... with respect to consequences which may result from the use of the articles to which the labeling or advertising relates under the conditions of use prescribed in the labeling or advertising thereof or under such conditions of use as are customary or usual."[7] Information accompanying prescription medications is specifically described as false or misleading if it omits the name and address of the dispenser, the serial number and date of the prescription, the name of the prescriber and patient, or any directions for use and cautionary statements.[8] Other material facts related to prescription medications are described in regulations promulgated by the U.S. Food and Drug Administration, which add that any drug labeling that furnishes or purports to furnish information for use, or which prescribes, recommends or suggests a dosage for the use of the drug,[9] must contain specific elements of information, unless clearly inapplicable, including:

1. a description of the drug, including
   a) the proprietary name and the established name of the drug, if any,
   b) the type of dosage form and the route of administration, and
   c) qualitative and/or quantitative ingredient information;
2. a concise factual summary of the clinical pharmacology and actions of the drug in humans;
3. the drug's indications and usage;
4. the drug's contraindications, including situations in which the drug should not be used because the risk of use clearly outweighs any possible benefit;
5. statements of
   a) warning concerning serious adverse reactions and potential safety hazards,
   b) limitations in use imposed by them, and
   c) steps that should be taken if they occur;
6. precautions to be taken including information regarding any special care to be exercised for safe and effective use of the drug, e.g., precautions concerning driving or the concomitant use of other substances that may have harmful additive effects;
7. information concerning adverse reactions reasonably associated with the use of the drug;
8. the types of abuse that can occur with the drug and the adverse reactions pertinent to them, including
   a) identification of susceptible patient populations,
   b) a description of the characteristic effects resulting from both psychological and physical dependence that occur with the drug, and
   c) an identification of the quantity of the drug over a period of time that may lead to tolerance or dependence, or both;
9. the signs, symptoms, and laboratory findings of acute overdosage and the general principles of treatment;
10. information concerning dosage and administration, including
    a) the recommended usual dose,
    b) the usual dosage range,
    c) if appropriate, an upper limit beyond which safety and effectiveness have not been established,
    d) the intervals recommended between doses,
    e) the usual duration of treatment, and
    f) any modification of dosage needed in special patient populations; and
11. any special handling and storage conditions.[1][10]

---

[1] Many states also require specific content to be included on prescription medication labeling. For example, California prohibits pharmacies from dispensing prescription medication unless the medication is

Penalties for violating the federal misbranding prohibition range from 1 year imprisonment and a $1,000 fine to 3 years imprisonment and a $10,000 fine.[11] At the same time, many states subject pharmacies and pharmacists to licensure discipline in cases where they are judged guilty of misbranding.[12]

1.2. The Obligation to Affix the Information to the Product

Another important requirement designed to protect the health and welfare of prescription medication consumers is the requirement that pharmacies securely affix certain basic information to the prescription medication containers they dispense to customers. At least 31 state legislatures and the District of Columbia have enacted such a requirement.[13] The obvious benefit of the requirement is to help prevent medication errors such as the accidental consumption of the wrong prescription medication.

The fact that certain basic information is required to be securely attached or affixed to prescription medications may be taken for granted by most pharmacy customers. And in the past, when no effective auxiliary communication of this information was either available or offered to the blind and visually-impaired, the requirement was largely irrelevant to this segment of the population. However, now that effective auxiliary communication aids for blind and visually-impaired medication users are available, which themselves can be securely affixed to prescription containers, the requirement to affix has new meaning, purpose and ability to benefit this particular segment of the population, whose desire to live an independent life and be able to care for themselves is the same as the rest of the population.

In summary, the regulatory requirements governing written information accompanying prescription medications, both in terms of the content required and the requirement to physically affix or attach such content to prescription containers, serve to protect an important public health interest: to help ensure the safe and effective use of prescription drug products. The inability of a significant segment of the population to read these written materials due to blindness and visual impairment,[2] and the public health disadvantage at which this population segment is placed due to their disability, has led to the development of relatively inexpensive, effective, easy-to-use, assistive technologies designed to communicate essential written drug information to the blind and visually-impaired in a way in which they can understand. What remains, however, in order for the blind and visually-impaired to benefit from these assistive technologies, is for pharmacies to acknowledge their ability and obligation to implement them.

---

correctly labeled with all of the following elements of information: (i) manufacturer's trade name of the drug, generic name and the name of the manufacturer or principal active ingredients, (ii) directions for the use of the drug, (iii) name of the patient and prescriber, (iv) date of issue, (v) name and address of the pharmacy, (vi) prescription number or other means of identifying the prescription, (vii) strength and quantity of the drug, (viii) expiration date of the effectiveness of the drug, (ix) condition for which the drug was prescribed and (x) commencing January 1, 2006 with certain exceptions, the physical description of the dispensed medication, including its color, shape, and any identification code that appears on the tablets or capsules. Cal. Bus. & Prof. Code 4076(a).

[2] For purposes of this article, blind and visually-impaired refers to those with visual impairments severe enough that they are unable to read large print materials.

2. Americans with Disabilities Act (ADA)

According to Title III of the Americans with Disabilities Act, an individual may not be discriminated against, on the basis of disability, in the full and equal enjoyment of the goods, services, facilities, privileges, advantages, or accommodations of any place of public accommodation.[14] Pharmacies are specifically listed in the ADA as public accommodations that must comply with this mandate.[15]

2.1. Auxiliary Communication Aids

Discrimination under the ADA includes a pharmacy's failure to take such steps as may be necessary to ensure that blind and visually-impaired individuals are not treated differently than sighted individuals because of the absence of auxiliary aids and services.[14] Federal regulations implementing the ADA further explain that auxiliary aids and services must be furnished by pharmacies where necessary to ensure effective communication with disabled individuals, including the blind and visually-impaired.[16] The term "auxiliary aids and services" is defined to specifically include qualified readers, taped texts, audio recordings, Brailled materials, large print materials, or other effective methods of making visually delivered materials available to individuals with visual impairments.[16] The term also includes the acquisition or modification of equipment or devices and other similar services and actions.[16]

Under the ADA, the type of auxiliary aid or service necessary to ensure effective communication will vary in accordance with the length and complexity of the communication involved. The U.S. Department of Justice instructs pharmacies to consult with their blind and visually-impaired customers wherever possible to determine what type of auxiliary aid is needed to ensure effective communication.[3][17] Furthermore, the ADA's standard prohibiting discrimination in the full and equal enjoyment of pharmacy goods, services and advantages would indicate that if an effective, auxiliary communication aid is available that can be securely affixed to prescription containers, as described above, that communication aid is to be preferred over those potential aids that are not capable of being securely affixed to prescription containers.

2.2. Exceptions to Pharmacy ADA Compliance

Pharmacies are allowed to forgo provision of auxiliary aids and services to their blind and visually-impaired customers only if they are able to demonstrate that taking such steps would fundamentally alter the nature of the good, service, facility, privilege, advantage, or that the accommodation being offered or would result in an undue burden on the pharmacy.[14] However, even if provision of a particular auxiliary aid or service by a pharmacy, brailled materials for example, were to result in a fundamental alteration or an undue burden, the pharmacy is still required to provide an alternative auxiliary aid or service, if one exists, that would not result in a fundamental alteration or undue burden.[16]

---

[3] The Department of Justice provides the example of a theater providing a blind or visually-impaired individual with a tape-recorded version of its printed program as an effective communication of the contents of the program.

According to the federal regulations implementing the ADA, the term fundamental alteration is defined as a modification so significant that it alters the essential nature of the goods, services, facilities, privileges, advantages, or accommodations offered.[17] An undue burden, on the other hand, is equivalent to the term "significant difficulty or expense."[4][16]

2.2.1. The Undue Burden Standard

Among the factors to be considered in determining whether an action would result in an undue burden are the following:

1. The nature and cost of the action;
2. The overall financial resources of the site or sites involved; the number of persons employed at the site; the effect on expenses and resources; legitimate safety requirements necessary for safe operation, including crime prevention measures; or any other impact of the action on the operation of the site;
3. The geographic separateness, and the administrative or fiscal relationship of the site or sites in question to any parent corporation or entity;
4. If applicable, the overall financial resources of any parent corporation or entity; the overall size of the parent corporation or entity with respect to the number of its employees; the number, type, and location of its facilities; and
5. If applicable, the type of operation or operations of any parent corporation or entity, including the composition, structure, and functions of the workforce of the parent corporation or entity.[17]

2.2.2. Comparing the Undue Burden Standard for Provision of Auxiliary Communication Aids to the Readily Achievable Standard for Barrier Removal

According to the Department of Justice (DOJ), the undue burden standard requires a greater level of effort by a public accommodation in providing auxiliary aids and services than does the readily achievable standard found in Title III of the ADA for removing barriers in existing facilities. Although "readily achievable" is therefore a lesser standard, the factors to be considered in determining what is readily achievable are identical to those listed above for determining undue burden.[5][17] Regulations issued by the DOJ contain a list of 21 examples of modifications that may be readily achievable.[17],[18] Among the examples provided are modifications that may be considered more difficult and costly to achieve than a pharmacy's provision of effective, auxiliary aids for the benefit of their blind and visually-impaired customers:

1. Installing wheelchair ramps;
2. Making curb cuts in sidewalks and entrances;
3. Installing flashing alarm lights;

---

[4] The definition of undue burden is identical to the definition of undue hardship used in Title I of the ADA as the limitation on an employer's obligation to reasonably accommodate an applicant or employee.

[5] Note that section III-4.4200 of the Technical Assistance Manual adds: "If the public accommodation is a facility that is owned or operated by a parent entity that conducts operations at many different sites, the public accommodation must consider the resources of both the local facility and the parent entity to determine if removal of a particular barrier is 'readily achievable.' The administrative and fiscal relationship between the local facility and the parent entity must also be considered in evaluating what resources are available for any particular act of barrier removal."

4. Widening doors;
5. Removing high pile, low density carpeting; and
6. Installing vehicle hand controls.

2.2.3. Availability of Tax Credit to Reduce ADA Compliance Burden

The already insignificant initial expense that may be incurred by pharmacies in implementing certain effective, auxiliary communication aids for the blind and visually-impaired is further diminished by a tax credit of up to $5,000 available to assist businesses in the purchase of effective auxiliary communication equipment for the benefit of the blind and visually-impaired. The tax credit, established under § 44 of the Internal Revenue Code, was created specifically to help businesses cover ADA-related expenditures.[6][19] Among the examples of expenditures covered by the credit are expenditures made or incurred:

1. for the purpose of removing communication barriers,
2. to provide qualified readers, taped texts, and other effective methods of making visually delivered materials available to individuals with visual impairments,
3. to acquire equipment or devices for individuals with disabilities, and
4. to provide other similar services, modifications, materials, or equipment.

Thus, pharmacies are required by law to furnish appropriate auxiliary aids and services where necessary to ensure effective communication with their blind and visually-impaired customers. While this requirement is to be balanced against any "undue burden" or "fundamental alteration" experienced by pharmacies, it is apparent that certain effective auxiliary communication aids available on the market today are less expensive and have less impact on pharmacy operations than the established practice of removing certain physical barriers for the benefit of customers who live with other types of disabilities. Furthermore, many pharmacies are entitled to take advantage of a significant tax credit specifically designed to encourage the implementation of effective auxiliary communication aids for the benefit of blind and visually-impaired customers. In any event, the Americans with Disabilities Act is not the only federal law addressing the obligation of pharmacies to provide their blind and visually-impaired customers with communications concerning prescription medication information by other means.

3. Health Insurance Portability and Accountability Act (HIPAA)

Health care providers considered to be "covered entities" according to privacy regulations promulgated pursuant to the Health Insurance Portability and Accountability Act (HIPAA) are required to permit individuals to request that communications of "protected health information" (PHI) from the health care provider be made by alternative means or at alternative locations. While health care providers

---

[6] A business that for the previous tax year had either revenues of $1,000,000 or less or 30 or fewer full-time workers is able to take advantage of this credit. For 2004, the appropriate form to use in claiming the credit was 2004 IRS Form 8826.

may require that such requests be made in writing, reasonable requests must be accommodated.[7][20]

3.1. Pharmacies are "covered entities" obligated to comply with HIPAA.

The term covered entity under HIPAA includes health care providers who transmit any health information in electronic form in connection with a transaction covered by the Health Insurance Portability and Accountability Act. The term healthcare provider includes entities that furnish, bill for or are paid for health care in the normal course of business, and the term health care includes the sale or dispensing of a drug, device, equipment or other item in accordance with a prescription.[21] Thus, pharmacies are covered entities obligated to comply with HIPAA privacy regulations.

3.2. Prescription information is "protected health information" under HIPAA.

Protected health information, the use and disclosure of which is regulated by HIPAA privacy regulations, means individually identifiable health information that is transmitted by or maintained in electronic or other forms of media.[21] Individually identifiable health information is health information created or received by a health care provider, including demographic information collected from an individual, which

1. identifies the individual or with respect to which there is a reasonable basis to believe the information can be used to identify the individual, and
2. relates to
   a) the past, present, or future physical or mental health or condition of the individual,
   b) the provision of health care to the individual, or
   c) the past, present, or future payment for the provision of health care to an individual.[21]

3.3. A blind or visually-impaired customer's request to receive communication of prescription label information via an auxiliary communication aid, as opposed to utilizing a family member as a reader, is reasonable

There are many valid reasons an individual may request PHI communications to be made by alternative means, including for example, the desire to prevent family members from learning about a particular treatment and the fear that all or part of the protected health information could subject the individual to abuse.[22] In its commentary concerning the HIPAA privacy rules, the U.S. Department of Health and Human Services (DHHS) has stated that a covered health care provider is not permitted to refuse to accommodate such a request based on its perception of the merits of the individual's reason for making the request. In fact, DHHS stated that a covered health care provider is not permitted to require the individual to provide a reason for the request as a condition of accommodating the request.[22]

---

[7] The two conditions a pharmacist may place on the provision of an alternative means accommodation are (i) information concerning how payment for pharmaceuticals will be handled; and, if applicable, (ii) specification of an alternative address or method of contacting the individual.

3.4. Communicating prescription label information via a privacy enabled auxiliary communication aid ensures that blind and visually-impaired individuals are able to exercise confidentiality rights they otherwise would may not be able to exercise

As stated by Rebecca Criswell of the Iowa Department for the Blind, "Currently, the only viable alternative is for the [blind or visually-impaired] individual to relinquish control over his or her medication to someone else such as another family member, a friend, or a paid in-home health provider. Obviously, this creates a dependency on others for care that is critical to one's good health and well-being, and individuals who were accustomed to being self-sufficient are given another reason to feel both diminished and vulnerable." However, the HIPAA privacy rules are designed to protect the right of an individual to not have his or her private health-related information disclosed to others, even family members if such a level of privacy is desired by the individual.

According to the rules, where a customer presents himself at a pharmacy and has the capacity to make health care decisions on his own behalf, the pharmacy is allowed to disclose the customer's PHI to the family members or close personal friends of the customer only if one of three conditions have been satisfied:

1. the pharmacy obtains the customer's agreement;
2. the pharmacy provides the customer with the opportunity to object to the disclosure, and the customer does not express an objection; or
3. the pharmacy reasonably infers from the circumstances, based on the exercise of professional judgment, that the customer does not object to the disclosure.

Unfortunately, even though pharmacy customers have the right to have their personal health information protected from disclosure to family and friends, according to comments received by the Food and Drug Administration during its Study on Making Prescription Pharmaceutical Information Accessible for Blind and Visually-Impaired Individuals, mandated by the Medicare Prescription Drug, Improvement, and Modernization Act of 2003,[23] blind and visually-impaired pharmaceutical users do not believe they are able to object to such a disclosure because they have no meaningful alternative to relying on their family members or friends to read the prescription label and insert describing the medication, usage and side effects on their behalf. However, certain auxiliary communication aids now on the market which are specifically designed for blind and visually-impaired pharmacy customers are providing such customers, for the first time, a meaningful opportunity to enjoy the ability to keep their prescription medication information private.

4. The Effectiveness of Currently Available Auxiliary Communication Aids and their Impact on the Pharmacies that Provide Them

Any available auxiliary communication aide should be judged from at least two perspectives: the effectiveness of the aide to the prescription medication user and the impact of providing the aide on pharmacy operations. With respect to the effectiveness of the aide to the prescription medication user, consideration should be given to:

1. the ability of the aide to communicate information completely,
2. the integrity of the information being communicated,
3. the ease of use, or user-friendliness, of the aide,
4. the ability of the user to access the information repeatedly,
5. the ability of the aid to be securely affixed to prescription containers, and
6. the ability of the aide or service to preserve the customer's privacy.

With respect to the impact of providing the aide on pharmacy operations, consideration should be given to:

a. the nature of the pharmacy action,
b. the initial cost of implementing the auxiliary aid or service,
c. the portability of the information from the pharmacy or pharmacist to the customer or the auxiliary aide,
d. the ongoing effect of providing the auxiliary aid or service on the pharmacy's expenses and resources, and
e. any other impact on the pharmacy.

Table 1 provides a summary of both traditional and recently developed methods of attempting to communicate prescription medication information to the blind and visually-impaired. These methods are judged against the specific elements of communication effectiveness and pharmacy impact issues described above.

Table 1. Available Auxiliary Communication Aids: Communication Effectiveness and Pharmacy Impact Issues

		Face-to-Face	Braille	Voice Cassette	Text-to-Speech CDs	Voice APLS	Text-to-Speech APLS/RFID
Communication Effectiveness Issues	**Information Completeness**	variable based on counselor	yes	variable based on counselor	yes	basic info	basic info
	Information Integrity	variable based on counselor	verification problematic	variable based on reader	consistent and verifiable	variable based on reader	consistent and verifiable
	User Friendliness	customer must rely on memory	usable by only 10% of the affected population	increasing difficulty w/ multiple medications	increasing difficulty w/ multiple medications	good	good
	Repeatability	problematic	yes	yes	yes	yes	yes
	Ability to Affix	no	no	no	no	limited to common sized pill bottles	yes
	Privacy Protection	only on-site at pharmacy	yes	yes	yes	yes	yes
Pharmacy Impact Issues	**Nature of Pharmacy Action**	some level typically provided already	easy to send information to printer	equivalent to face-to-face counseling	moderate software difficulties	equivalent to face-to-face counseling	easy to send information to RFID label printer
	Initial Cost of Pharmacy Action	none	expensive	low	low	low	moderate
	Information Portability	problematic	good	problematic	moderate software difficulty	problematic	good
	Ongoing Effect on Expenses and Resources	insignificant if brief	insignificant	insignificant if brief	insignificant	moderate	insignificant

4.1. Face to Face Counseling

Face-to-face counseling is currently the most commonly used form of auxiliary communication or service. However, it is also one of the most ineffective.

Commentary received by the U.S. Department of Health and Human Services during its "Study on How to Make Prescription Pharmaceutical Information, Including Drug Labels and Usage Instructions, Accessible for Blind and Visually-impaired Individuals" (hereinafter referred to as the "DHHS Accessibility Study") indicates that the most common alternative method of communicating written prescription medication information to the blind and visually-impaired is in the form of a verbal explanation from a pharmacist to the customer or to a friend or family member of the customer.[24] While some form of face-to-face, verbal counseling is provided in nearly all pharmacies today and the impact of such communications on pharmacies' initial and ongoing operations can be insignificant if the communications are brief, the effectiveness of relying on face-to-face, verbal communications as an effective auxiliary communication aide to the blind and visually-impaired is questionable.

A brief verbal counseling session would not typically provide the customer with <u>complete</u> medication information, as described above and mandated by some states and the FDA. And while a complete communication of the written information is possible, the impact to pharmacies on expenses and resources rises in relation to the amount of time spent in face-to-face counseling sessions. In fact, comments received over the course of the DHHS Accessibility Study reported that those providing drug information are often too busy to provide sufficient verbal counseling or information.[24] Thus, there is predictably a wide degree of vulnerability in the completeness of the information communicated by pharmacies in verbal counseling sessions. One of the primary reasons for legal mandates governing the content of prescription labeling again becomes apparent. An incomplete communication is not an effective communication.

During face-to-face counseling, customer privacy concerns may be addressed by pharmacies by implementing safeguards such as speaking to the customer in an area separate from other waiting customers or asking the other waiting customers to keep an appropriate distance from counters used for patient counseling. However, while customers are able to enjoy their privacy rights in face-to-face verbal counseling sessions, problems remain with respect to issues such as user-friendliness and information integrity, repeatability and portability.

Whether the verbal communication is brief or extensive, the integrity of the communication is as variable as the reading and speaking skills of the thousands of pharmacists and pharmacy technicians delivering the communication. Such a wide variety in reading and speaking skills increases the potential for miscommunication, including mispronunciations, omissions and erroneous statements. Such faulty communications are not effective.

With respect to user-friendliness, blind and visually-impaired pharmacy customers are forced to rely on their memory of the verbal communication. Such a reliance on the customer's ability to later recall complex information received from a verbal explanation is predictably problematic, especially considering that the customer may be taking numerous prescription medications simultaneously. The risk of memory failure leading to adverse health consequences rises in relation to the amount of time having transpired since the verbal explanation and in relation to the number of prescription medications being utilized by the blind or visually-impaired customer. For the customer to be forced to return to the pharmacy for numerous repeat face-to-face verbal communications only further increases the burden of this method of auxiliary communication on both the customer and the pharmacy.

4.2. Braille Embossers/Printers

Braille printers, also called embossers, have mixed communication effectiveness and a mixed impact on pharmacies. The printers have the capability of printing complete medication information, and the difference to a pharmacist or pharmacy technician of sending information to an ordinary printer versus sending information to a braille printer is insignificant. Those pharmacy customers who are able to read braille are able to read the printouts repeatedly and are able to keep the printouts private in the same manner that sighted pharmacy customers are able to keep ordinary written medication information private. However, there are several significant problems associated with the utilization of braille as an auxiliary communication aid.

One of the biggest problems with braille as an auxiliary communication aid is that only a small percentage of the blind and visually-impaired population (approximately 10%) are able to read it, primarily those who became blind in early life. The vast majority of older blind and visually-impaired individuals do not know braille.[24] In addition, very few pharmacists would be able to read the braille printout in order to confirm the accuracy of the medication information produced.[24] Another significant problem with utilizing braille printers as an auxiliary communication aid is their impact to pharmacies in terms of cost. According to the American Foundation for the Blind, "the price of a braille printer is directly related to the volume of braille production required—between $1,800 and $5,000 for smaller volume production and between $10,000 and $80,000 for larger volume production."[25] Finally, braille printouts containing even basic information are known to be particularly bulky or large, and pharmacies would find it difficult if not impossible to securely affix more than a few words of brailled prescription medication information on a small prescription container.

4.3. Cassette, Human Voice Recording

Speaking medication information into a cassette recorder is similar to face-to-face counseling in many respects. The nature of the pharmacy action, the ongoing effect of the action on the pharmacy's expenses and resources, and issues involving information portability, integrity and completeness are virtually identical. To illustrate, there is little difference between a pharmacy or pharmacy technician reading medication information into a recorder versus reading the information directly to the pharmacy customer. Brief verbal communications are typically provided already at most pharmacies across the United States. However, dictating comprehensive medication can result in undesired, lengthy interruptions of pharmacy operations. Therefore, information communicated via cassette recordings may tend to be incomplete, the extent of the incompleteness being related to the pharmacist's or pharmacy technician's perceived need to attend to other pharmacy matters. The integrity of the information communicated is also questionable due to pharmacists' and pharmacy technicians' variable reading and speaking skills, leading to an increased potential for miscommunication, including mispronunciations, omissions and erroneous statements.

Unlike face-to-face counseling, however, pharmacies do incur a small initial cost to implement cassette recording as an auxiliary communication aid. The initial cost of a cassette recording device is between $15 to $550, depending on the type of device and manufacturer. Handheld microcassette recorders are priced from $15[8] to $300,[9] while microcassette transcribers are priced from $200[10] to $550.[11] Microcassettes with a recording time of 60 minutes cost approximately $1 to $1.50 each.

Cassette recordings containing complete medication information offer blind and visually-impaired pharmacy customers the option to receive the communication repeatedly and privately. However, because the cassette recording is likely to contain only basic medication information, the customer would need to either return to the pharmacy for more complete information or possibly sacrifice desired privacy by relying on friends, family members or others to read the information.

In addition, the benefits gained by requiring that medication information be physically and securely affixed or attached to prescription containers is lost with the cassette recording method, which inherently requires the ability to place the cassette into a cassette player. Blind and visually-impaired pharmacy customers taking

---

[8] COBY CX R122 Microcassette Dictaphone.

[9] Dictaphone Voice Processor Microcassette Dictation Recorder.

[10] Sony M2000 Microcassette Transcriber.

[11] Voice Solutions DA-116 Universal Deluxe Digital Transcriber Dictaphone.

multiple prescription medications risk mismatching a particular cassette recording with the drug it relates to.

4.4. Text-to-Audio Software and CD Writer Combination

Another potential auxiliary communication aid pharmacies may implement is a combination of text-to-audio software and a compact disc (CD) writer. This method of communication offers information completeness, integrity, portability, repeatability and privacy. However, the initial and ongoing cost and impact of this solution on any given pharmacy depends largely on information technology support available to the pharmacy or the level of information technology skills possessed by existing pharmacy staff. At the same time, the CD recording method of communication suffers the same flaw as cassette recordings in terms of the inability of both methods to ensure that important medication information be physically and securely affixed to the prescription containers they contain information about.

Text-to-audio programs range in price from $25[12] to $70,[13] and compact disc writers range from $20[14] to $685.[15] After properly installing the hardware and software on an existing computer, medication information data residing on the computer is converted by the text-to-audio software to an audio format such as MP3. The MP3 audio file is then written onto a compact disc which is given to the blind or visually-impaired customer, who is then able to listen to the medication information on any compact disc player supporting the MP3 format.

Technical difficulties encountered with do-it-yourself software and hardware installation and operation, however, may have a negative impact on pharmacies. For example, cursory reviews of compact disc writer support websites reveal problems such as (i) errors occurring resulting in termination of the installation process, (ii) drive letters not recognized, (iii) the CD writer not recognizing the media inserted into the drive, (iv) the burn process apparently completing coupled with no data being written to the disc, and (v) numerous other technical error messages. As an alternative to self help trouble shooting, pharmacies may conclude that third-party technical support availability is required.

Thus, the costs associated with such third-party technical support may result in a negative impact to ongoing expenses and resources as a result of implementing the text-to-audio and CD writer combination as an auxiliary communication aid solution.

4.5. Audible Prescription Labeling Systems

Fortunately, technological advances in recent years have enabled the development of new types of auxiliary communication aids which overcome many of the limitations inherent in traditional types of aids. Audible Prescription Labeling Systems (APLS) are relatively new developments designed specifically to address prescription medication information concerns involving blind and visually-impaired pharmacy

---

[12] Alive Text to Speech v5.2.1.0 by Alive Media.

[13] Text-to-Audio v7.0 by Premier Assistive.

[14] Norcent RW-532 CD-RW IDE drive.

[15] Plextor PlexWriter Premium CD-RW IDE drive.

customers. Four APLS technologies have been marketed in the U.S. since 2000,[16][24] one of which combines radio frequency identification (RFID) technology with text-to-speech capabilities to create the most effective auxiliary communication aid available on the market today. While each of the APLS communication aids have a relatively insignificant impact on pharmacy expenses and operations, they do vary in communication effectiveness.

Three of the four available APLS aids rely on human voice recordings[17] which, as described above in relation to face-to-face counseling and cassette recordings, pose problems with respect to information completeness, integrity and portability due to pharmacists' and pharmacy technicians' time restraints and variable reading and communication skills. These three also are further limited to prescription medications packaged in standard-sized prescription vials (i.e., pill bottles) and are not functional for use with other commonly used prescription medication packaging such as odd-shaped glass and plastic bottles (for example, dropper bottles and oval-shaped cough medicine bottles), blister packs and boxes.

One of the four available APLS communication aids on the market overcomes issues related to information integrity and portability by utilizing text-to-speech technology.[18] This aid also utilizes an RFID enabled label that securely affixes to any type of prescription medication container, including odd-shaped glass and plastic bottles, blister packs and boxes. Pharmacists or pharmacy technicians pass textual prescription medication information from their computer to a dedicated, small-footprint RFID label printer which encodes the prescription information in an electronic format on a microchip embedded in the label. In the home, the patient uses a hand-held reader, which decodes the label information using speech synthesis technology, to hear medication information such as patient name, drug name and dosage information, instructions for use, warnings and cautions, the prescription number and the name and phone number of the pharmacy and the prescribing doctor.

Unlike face-to-face counseling, the utilization of text-to-speech APLS aids takes a minimal amount of pharmacy time, and the integrity of the communication is ensured because the variable communication skills of pharmacists and technicians are not being relied upon. Furthermore, the information is easily repeatable, so there is no excessive need for the blind or visually-impaired customer to rely upon their memory. In addition, unlike braille embossed medication information sheets, text-to-speech APLS communications are able to be understood by the vast majority of blind and visually-impaired pharmacy customers, and unlike cassette and CD recordings, RFID labels used by text-to-speech APLS systems are able to be securely affixed to, and do not need to be removed from, prescription medication containers.

---

[16] The four products identified are (i) En-Vision America's ScripTalk, (ii) MedivoxRx Technologies, Inc.'s Rex Disposable Talking Bottle, (iii) TalkingRx, Inc.'s Talking Rx and (iv) ASKO Corporation's Aloud Audio Labeling System.

[17] The products made by MedivoxRx, TalkingRx and ASKO rely on human voice recording.

[18] En-Vision America's ScripTalk.

5. Conclusion

While several methods of communicating prescription medication information to the blind and visually-impaired exist, the development of text-to-speech APLS systems utilizing RFID labels has now made it possible for pharmacies to effectively communicate such information to the blind and visually-impaired with minimal difficulty and expense and with insignificant alteration of the essential nature of pharmacy operations. In addition, thanks to these specially-designed systems, blind and visually-impaired pharmacy customers are now able to enjoy the same privacy rights enjoyed by sighted customers, rights which have historically been forfeited due to a lack of alternative means of receiving prescription medication communications. At the same time, pharmacies can be confident that their provision of text-to-speech APLS systems utilizing RFID labels is the most appropriate and cost-effective solution to compliance with numerous state and federal laws governing prescription medication information content, placement, privacy and non-discrimination in communications.

References

[1] John P. Santell, et al., *Medication Error Trends for 1999-2003*, 149(4) Drug Topics HSE22 (February 21, 2005).
[2] Committee on Quality of Health Care in America, Institute of Medicine, To Err is Human - Building a Safer Health System (1999). Retrieved from Institute of Medicine via http://www.iom.edu/includes/DBFile.asp?id=4117.
[3] Susan Camp and Rodney Hicks, *Medication Errors in the Patient's Home*, 148(8) Drug Topics HSE14 (April 19, 2004).
[4] U.S. Food and Drug Administration. Medication Errors. Retrieved from U.S. Food and Drug Administration via http://www.fda.gov/cder/handbook/mederror.htm.
[5] Pharmacists offer tips to help patients avoid medication errors, Patient Care Law Weekly, pg. 29, (August 21, 2005).
[6] Misbranded Drugs and Devices, 21 U.S.C. 352(a) (2005).
[7] Federal Food, Drug, and Cosmetic Act Definitions, 21 U.S.C. 321(n) (2004).
[8] Exemptions and Consideration for Certain Drugs, Devices, and Biological Products, 21 U.S.C. 353(b)(2) (2004).
[9] Prescription Drugs for Human Use, 21 C.F.R 201.100(d) (2002).
[10] General Requirements on Content and Format of Labeling for Human Prescription Drugs, 21 C.F.R. 201.56 (1979) and Specific Requirements on Content and Format of Labeling for Human Prescription Drugs, 21 C.F.R. 201.57 (1998).
[11] Federal, Food, Drug, and Cosmetic Act Penalties, 21 U.S.C. 333(a) (2003).
[12] General Operating Standards for Pharmacies, Code D.C. Mun. Reg. 22-1909.5 (1991), Counterfeit Drugs, Fla. Admin. Code 64B16-27.101 (1991), Drug Dispensing and Prescription Records, N.J. Admin. Code 13:39-7.18 (2005), and Grounds for Discipline for a Pharmacist License, 22 Tex. Admin. Code 281.7(a)(29)(A) (1998).
[13] Arkansas Uniform Narcotic Drug Act: Labels, Ark. Code Ann. § 20-64-210 (1947); Requirements for Prescriptions, Cal. Bus & Prof Code § 4076 (2004); Pharmaceutical Labeling, Colo. Rev. Stat. § 12-22-123 (2003); Labeling of Package or Container of Controlled Substances, Conn. Gen. Stat. § 21a-256 (1999); Pharmacy Labeling, Del. Code Ann. tit. 24, § 2536 (2005); Regulation of Manufacture, Distribution, and Dispensing of Prescriptions, D.C. Code Ann. § 48-903.08 (1981); Pharmacist's Dispensing Procedure, Fla. Stat. Ann. § 465.186 (1997); Pharmacist and Practitioner, Fla. Stat. Ann. § 893.04 (1999); Regulation of Manufacture, Distribution, and Dispensing of Prescriptions, Haw. Rev. Stat. § 329-38 (2003); Labels, Haw. Rev. Stat. §§ 329-39 (1996); Information Required on Label, Idaho Code § 37-2731 (1972); Pharmacists' Violations and Penalties, Idaho Code § 54-1732 (1985); The

Pharmacy Practice Act of 1987: Labeling, Ill. Rev. Stat. ch. 225, para. 85/22 (2005); Requirements for Dispensing Controlled Substances, Ill. Rev. Stat. ch. 720, para. 570/312 (2005); Indiana Legend Drug Act, Ind. Code Ann. § 16-42-19-11 (1999); Distribution by Practitioner or Pharmacist, Prescription Requirements: Penalties, Ky. Rev. Stat. Ann. § 218A.180 (1998); Louisiana Pharmacy Practice Acts Definitions, La. Rev. Stat. Ann. § 37:1164 (1999); Filling of Prescription and Required Information on Label, Mass. Gen. Laws Ann. ch. 94C, § 21 (1988); Delivery of Prescriptions, Mass. Gen. Laws Ann. ch. 94C, § 27 (1993); Labeling of Prescription Drug Containers, Minn. Stat. Ann. § 151.212 (1988); Labeling Requirements, Mo. Rev. Stat. § 195.100 (1998); How Prescriptions Must be Labeled, Mo. Rev. Stat. § 338.059 (1978); Labeling Requirements, Neb. Rev. Stat. § 28-415 (2001); Contents of Label on Drug Package, Nev. Rev. Stat. Ann. § 585.420 (1977); Requirements for Labeling Containers for Prescribed Drugs, Nev. Rev. Stat. Ann. § 639.2801 (2003); Prescription Labels, N.H. Rev. Stat. Ann. § 318:47-a (2002); Form of Label to be Used by Pharmacists, N.J. Stat. Ann. § 24:21-17 (1986); Prescription Requirements, N.J. Stat. Ann. § 45:14-15 (1991); Prescriptions, N.M. Stat. Ann. § 30-31-18 (2005); Prescriptions, N.Y. Educ. Law § 6810 (2003); Prescription Label Requirements, N.C. Gen. Stat. § 106-134.1 (1981); Labeling of Prescription Drugs, N.D. Cent. Code, § 19-02.1-14.1 (2001); Controlled Substances Labeling, Ohio Rev. Code Ann. § 3719.08 (1998); Dispensing Dangerous Drugs, Okl. Stat. Ann. tit. 59, § 355.1 (2005); Prescription Labels, Okl. Stat. Ann. tit. 63, § 2-314 (2005); Labeling Requirements, Or. Rev. Stat. § 689.505 (1993); Contents of Prescription Drug Label, Tex. Occ. Code § 567.001 (1999); Prescription Labels, Utah Code Ann. § 58-17b-602 (2004); Labeling of Regulated Drugs, Vt. Stat. Ann. tit. 18, § 4212 (1968); Prescription Drug Labeling Requirements, Wash. Rev. Code Ann. § 69.41.050 (2003); and Prescription Drugs and Prescription Devices, Wis. Stat. Ann. § 450.11 (2001).

[14] Prohibition of Discrimination by Public Accommodation, 42 U.S.C. 12182 (1990).

[15] Equal Opportunity for Individuals with Disabilities, Definitions Applicable to Public Accommodations and Services Operated by Private Entities, 42 U.S.C. 12181(7)(F) (1990).

[16] Auxiliary Aids and Services, 28 C.F.R. 36.303 (1991).

[17] Department of Justice, ADA Title III Technical Assistance Manual (2005).

[18] Removal of Barriers, 28 C.F.R. 36.304 (1991).

[19] Expenditures to Provide Access to Disabled Individuals, 26 U.S.C. § 44 (1990).

[20] Rights to Request Privacy Protection for Protected Health Information, 45 C.F.R. 164.522(b) (2002).

[21] HIPAA Security and Privacy General Definitions, 45 C.F.R. 160.103 (2002).

[22] Standards for Privacy of Individually Identifiable Health Information, 65 F.R. 82462, 82553 (Dec. 28, 2000).

[23] U.S. Food and Drug Administration. Docket 2004N-0221: Medicare Prescription Drug, Improvement, and Modernization Act of 2003 Section 107(F)B. Retrieved from U.S. Food and Drug Administration via http://www.fda.gov/ohrms/dockets/dockets/04n0221/04N0221.htm.

[24] Report to Congress, The Medicare Prescription Drug, Improvement, and Modernization Act of 2003, Section 107(f): A Study on How to Make Prescription Pharmaceutical Information, Including Drug Labels and Usage Instructions, Accessible for Blind and Visually-impaired Individuals, Department of Health and Human Services, May, 2005.

[25] American Federation for the Blind. Braille Technology. Retrieved from American Federation for the Blind via http://www.afb.org/Section.asp?SectionID=4&TopicID=31&DocumentID=1282.

Promoting Independence for Older Persons with Disabilities
W.C. Mann and A. Helal (Eds.)
IOS Press, 2006

An Ultrasonic Urine Sensor for Aged People

Hiroyuki KODAMA [a,1], Yu JING [a], Eiji IWATSUBO [b], Yasuo KUCHINOMACHI [c], Hisashi YOSHIMURAD [d], Naomi Kikuchi KUCHITSU [d]

[a] *Department for Human Science and Biomedical Engineering, Institute of Advanced Industrial Science and Technology, Tsukuba, Japan*
[b] *Labor Welfare Corporation, Spinal Injuries Center*
[c] *Shizuoka University of Welfare Faculty of Social Welfare, Yaidu, Japan*
[d] *Takeshiba Electric Co., Ltd. Kanagawa 3371-32, Japan*

Abstract. Urinary incontinence can impact independence and quality of life and is common among older persons. If the amount of urine can be predicted in advance, then it can help those with incontinence in discharging on time. To serve this purpose, we developed an ultrasonic urine sensor. This device is small in volume and light in weight, thus permitting easy access by people with incontinence.

Keywords. Urinary incontinence, bladder, urine, sensors

Introduction

Maintaining independence and active participation in society is something we all hope to attain. When encountered with the problem of urinary incontinence, freedom may be compromised. Nearly 5 percent of the world population suffers from urinary incontinence. Half of these people are over age 65. Urinary incontinence can cause depression and result in a decrease in social activities. If the amount of urine can be ascertained in advance, then accidents may be avoided. This could also reduce the burden for care providers. To address this problem, we have worked out an effective method for the prediction of urine accumulation in a bladder and developed an ultrasonic urine sensor.

The ultrasonic urine sensor is used to measure bladder volume by means of ultrasound employed outside the human body. It is based on the difference of sound impedance in the liquid within the bladder and tissue of human body. To detect the appropriate time for urine withdrawal, this device is small in volume, light in weight and inexpensive. In terms of the expansion characteristics of a bladder, a measurement index is devised and employed in the ultrasonic urine sensor. The measurements of a bladder volume and its internal pressure are conducted for some patients who had injuries in their spinal cords and for some patients who received regular inspections of urinary tract imaging. Comparisons are made between the predictions by the urine sensor, the amount of the physiology salt solution injected, and the amount of the urine withdrawal. The performance of the urine sensor is then highlighted.

1. Method of Prediction in the Ultrasonic Urination Sensor

The variation in the shape of bladder can be well observed with magnetic resonance imager (MRI) during urine accumulation. The patients were asked to lie on their backs with their abdomens in the center of a magnetic field of the MRI. The shape of bladders was then photographed at 30 min, 1 hr, 1.5 hrs and 2 hrs, respectively, after patients had just discharged their urine. In Fig.1 a bladder is identified to have expansions in the top part due to the accumulation of urine gradually, while there appears almost no shape change in other parts. [1]~[5]

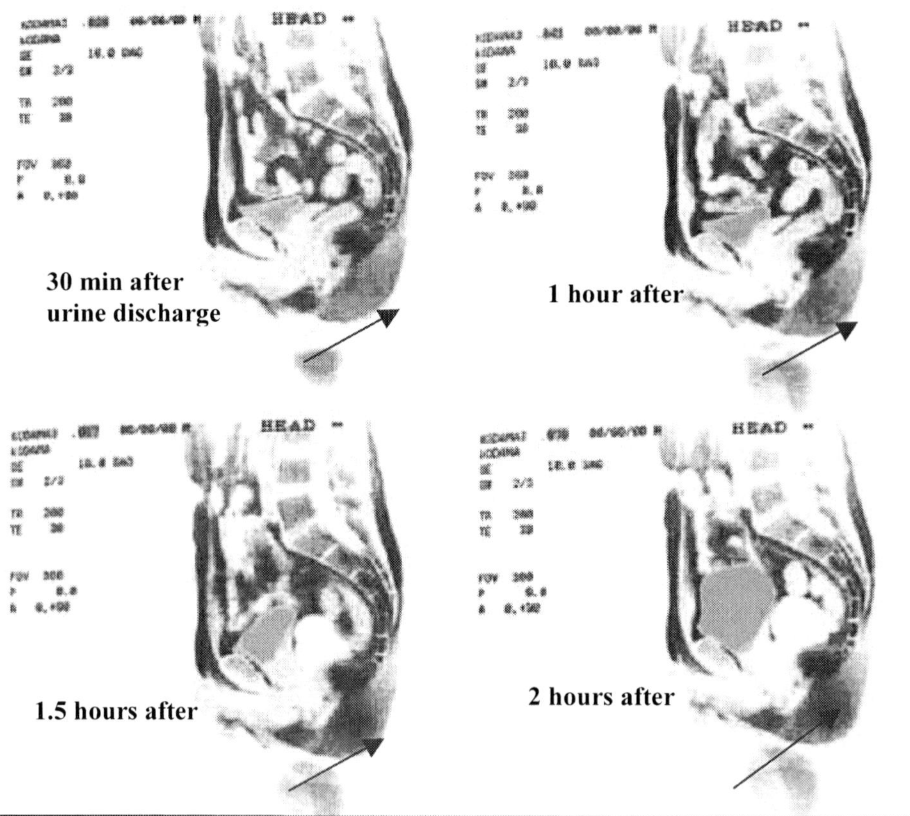

Figure 1. Expansion of the bladder on the urine accumulation observed by MRI. There is an expansion of the top part and almost no shape changes of bottom part.

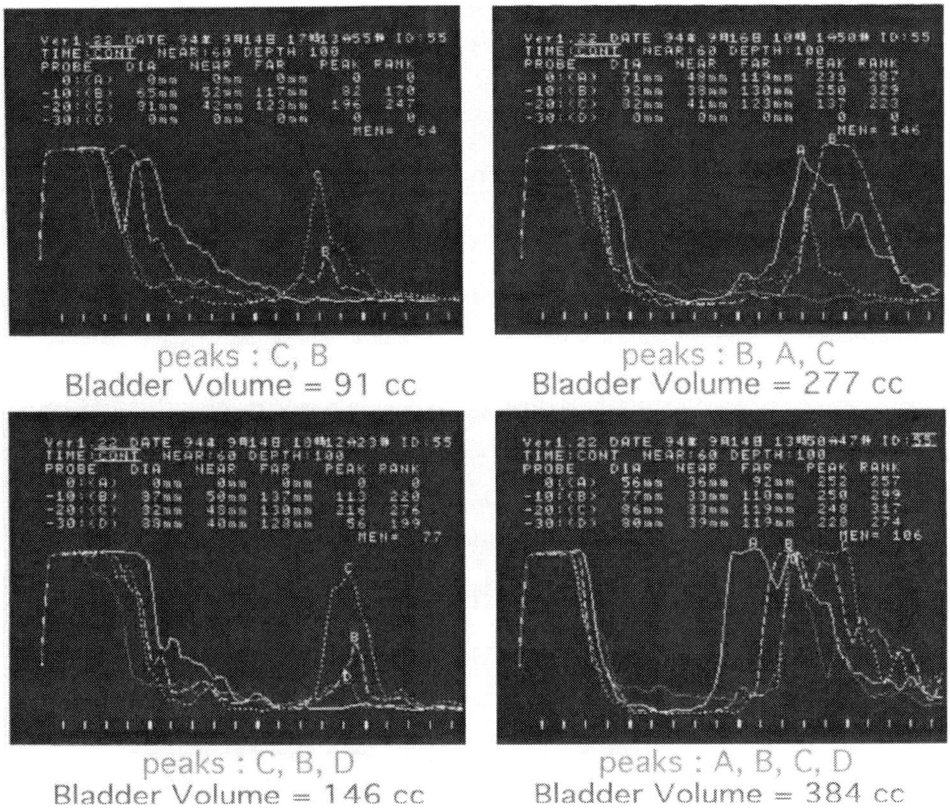

Figure 2. Increase of the number of piezoelectric elements embedded in a probe of the ultrasonic urination sensor, giving ultrasound echo signals from the bladder rear wall

The ultrasonic urination sensors adopts four piezoelectric elements embedded in a probe and arrayed on the cephalic direction, based on the bladder expansion characteristics. Upon urine accumulation, the number of elements in function is increased as is shown in Figure 2, giving ultrasound echo signals from the bladder rear wall ls from the bladder rear wall and thus the signal intensity is augmented. From these two features a measuring index of bladder expansion was devised as a summation of each element's front wall back, wall distance multiplied by back wall echo peak intensity. The principle of the ultrasonic urine sensor is well illustrated in Figure.3.

2. Results and Discussions

Clinical measurement was performed in three medical facilities. In the urology department of the hospital affiliated with the University of Tsukuba, simultaneous examination of urine flow dynamics (measuring pressure in a bladder, cystometry) and measurement of the amount of urine were carried out with 68 persons (42 men, 26 women) of 3-82 years-old. The correspondence data between the amount of physiological saline solution poured and the measurement index was acquired. In the

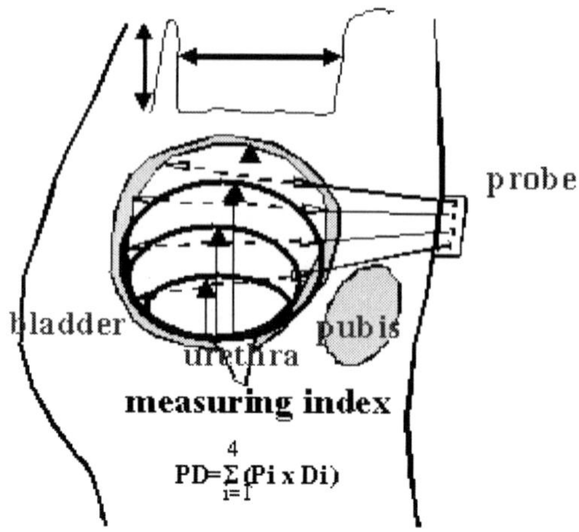

Figure 3. Principle of ultrasonic urination sensor and schematic illustration of expansion of the bladder

spinal injury center of Japan, same inspections were performed for patients with the cooperation of 23 persons (20 men, three women) aging from 14 to 74 years old. Moreover, experimental tests were conducted in the Institute of Advanced Industrial and Science and Technology of Japan (AIST). Persons in normal health were included in the tests during this experimental evaluation, including 4 men and 5 women. A total of 13 measurements were conducted.

Figures 4 and 5 show the test results conducted in the urology department of the hospital affiliated with the University of Tsukuba and the spinal injuries center of Japan. Linear correspondence was confirmed when the amount of injection was below 300ml. Over this value, although the bladder capacity increased, the index value seldom increased. To overcome the saturation problem, modifications are made on the design of the ultrasonic urination sensor. Figure 6 shows the test results in the AIST. As can be seen, even if the capacity is about 600ml, a direct proportion relationship has been maintained by the modified sensor with a large dynamic measurement range. This result indicated that the ultrasonic urination sensor could express the essentially accurate relationship with bladder capacity.

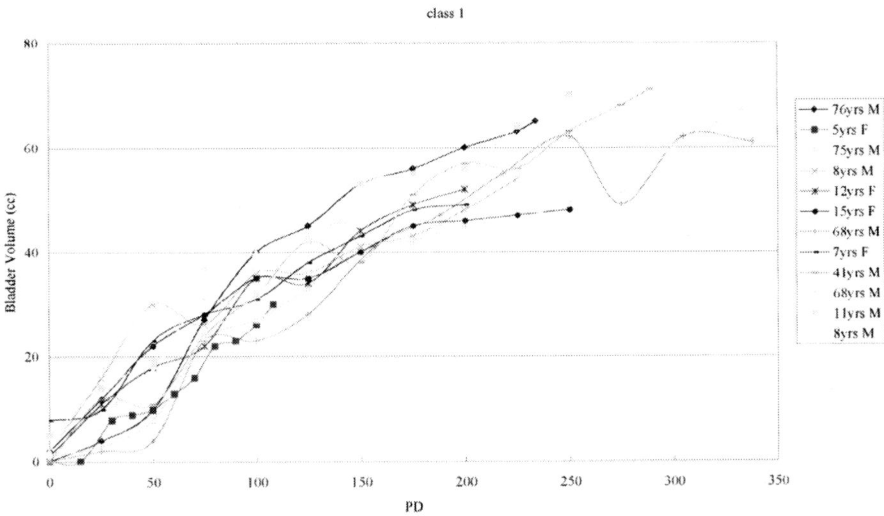

Figure 4. The results obtained in the urology department of the hospital affiliated with the University of Tsukuba

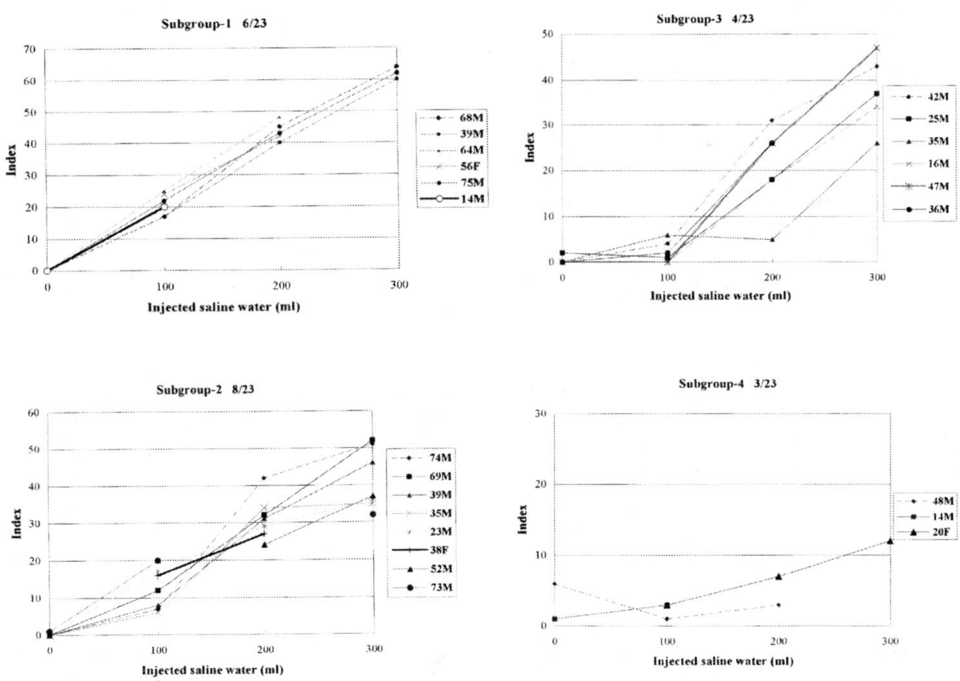

Figure 5. Various cases of index-injection relations

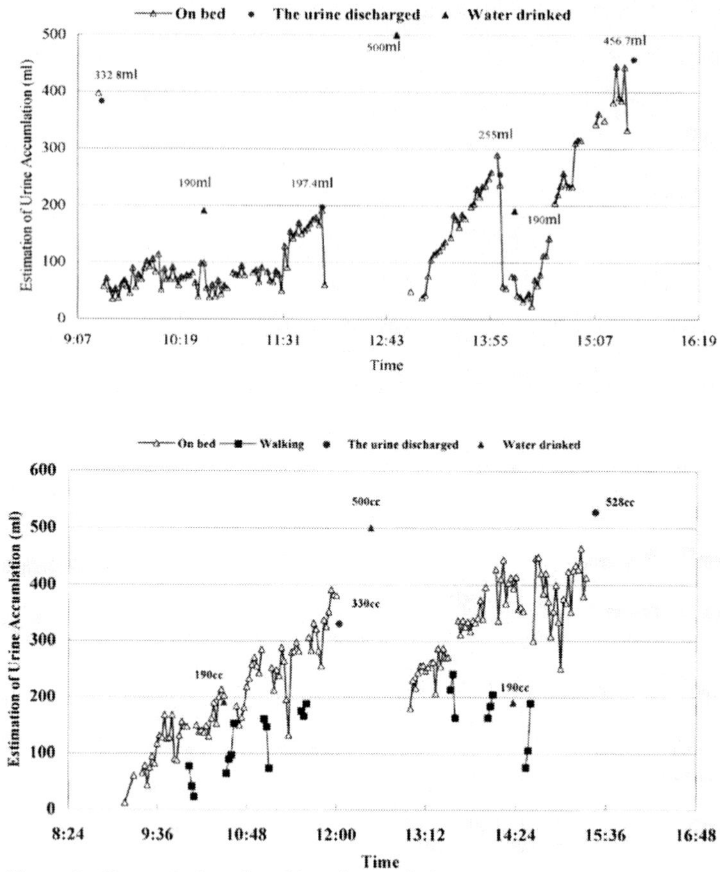

Figure.6. Two typical results of the urine predictions in AIST. 6-1. a man tested, 6-2. a woman tested

3. Commercialization and Potential Applications of the Ultrasonic Urine Sensor

The ultrasonic urination sensor has now received permission for medical use by the Welfare Ministry of Japan. Commercialization of the ultrasonic urine sensor has made significant progress currently. The ultrasonic urine sensor can now be made so small and light enough that it is very easy to fix it on the abdomens of patients (Figure 7). In fact, the portability and low price has made it possible to be accessed by various patients and medical centers.

The ultrasonic urine sensor has significant potential for wide use as a medical device in clinical treatment centers, nursery stations and homes. With the assistance of the sensor, users can be alerted to discharge before the bladder becomes full and accidental discharge occurs.

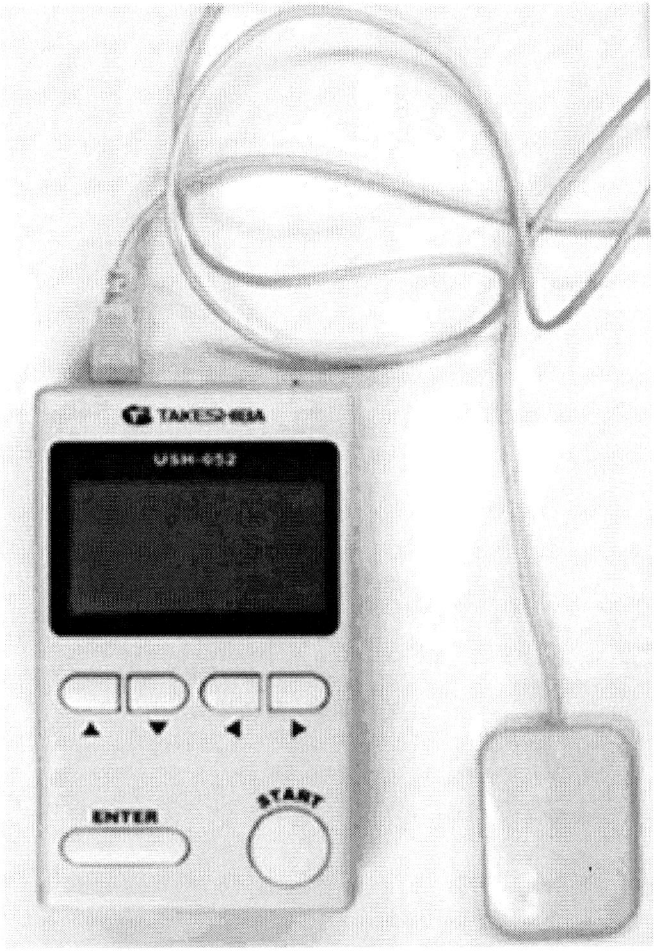

Figure 7. The ultrasonic urine sensor

4. Conclusions

The results of the clinical test are striking, as in all the experimental tests there exists a definite monotonic relationship between their bladder volumes and the corresponding sensor outputs. Based on these encouraging results, we reach a conclusion that the ultrasonic urine sensor can effectively reflect the expansion of bladders incurred by urine accumulation. It is strongly anticipated that the ultrasonic urine sensor can be used by those who suffer from urinary incontinence.

Acknowledgement

The authors are grateful to the valuable guidance of Prof. Wada of Hokkaido University during the design and development of the ultrasonic urine sensor.

References

[1] Hiroyuki Kodama, Hisashi Yoshimura, Jun Sugawara, Yoshihiko Nagata, Eiji Iwatsubo, Kiyomi Matsuo,Development Of A Wearable Ultrasonic Sensor For Urination Dysfunction, *International Ergonomics Assocation XVth Triennial Congress* August 24-29, 2003, Seoul, Korea

[2] Hiroyuki Kodama, Hisashi Yoshimura, Eiji Iwatsubo, Ultrasonic Urination Sensor For Spinal Cord Injured Aged People, *International Ergonomics Assocation XVth Triennial Congress* August 24-29, 2003, Seoul, Korea

[3] Kodama, H., Kuchinomachi, Y., Hieda, I., Yoshimura, H., Mizuno, K. and Nishimura, T. New Sensor for Prevention of Urinary Incontinence, *On Proceedings of the 4th Asia-Pacific Conference on Medical & Biological Engineering.* 309. 1999.

[4] Kodama, H., Kuchinomachi, Y., Yamauchi, Y., Hieda, I., Sato, S., Takeichi, H. and Matsumoto, H. Ultra sonic Urination Sensor for homeuse, *On IEA'97. Proceedings of the 13th Triennial Congress of the International Ergonomics Association,* 5, 582-584. 1997.

[5] Kodama, H., Hieda, I., Kuchinomachi, Y., Takeichi, H. and Matsumoto, H. Non-invasive Ultrasonic Urination Sensor for Ambulatory Patient Support *On Methods of Information in Medicine,* 33, 97-100. 1994.

Medication Reminding for Older Adults Using Personal Digital Assistants

Anthony A. STERNS [a,1], and Harvey L. STERNS [b]
[a]*Creative Action LLC, Akron, OH USA*
[b]*The University of Akron, Institute for Life-Span, Development and Gerontology, Department of Psychology, Akron, OH*

Abstract. Forty-six older adults (average age 72 years) were successfully trained to use personal digital assistant standard programs and a program called RxReminder for medication reminding. Successful usage was demonstrated through the use of several performance measures. The RxReminder interface is built on universal design principles and the guidelines for computer interfaces described by Czaja and Lee [1]. A pillbox that integrates onto the body of the PDA was also created as a place to store mid-day pills. Unlike the plastic weekly pillbox, the system provides alarms, a picture of the pill, dosage, warnings, doctor and pharmacy information, and a place for the pills themselves in a single location. Forty-two participants completed a 3-month use test of the device. A physical pill count was also conducted. Average compliance for pill taking while using the device was -.05 pills per month with two-thirds of the participants missing 1 pill or less in the third month of the study. The RxReminder interface received the highest usability rating and was significantly higher then several of the PDA standard applications.

Introduction

Recent studies discuss various medical applications for PDAs including drug references, diagnostic guides, "e-prescribing," medical calculators, toxicology references, patient tracking databases, and medical literature databases [2]. Recent conference papers have begun to report using PDAs and PDA devices for medical journaling and remote communication with physicians and other medical staff [3].

Medication-related problems represent a huge cost to the United States economy. Over $76 billion dollars are spent annually on medical complications caused by not taking medication appropriately. We believe the PDA has the potential to solve the problem of remembering to take medicine and provide many other benefits.

Reducing the barriers to using a PDA will increase the number of people who can benefit from the long list of features a PDA can offer. Our efforts included creating a curriculum targeted to older adults to teach PDA usage skills [4] as well as creating software with improved interface and operation [1]. We designed these modifications to lower the barriers required to use a PDA and to improve the likelihood of success for the participants.

Our research team felt it was important to link the reminder program and the medications. To accomplish this, we designed and manufactured a prototype PDA pillbox that integrates with the PDA and provides a compartment for a daily dosage of medications and supplements (see Figure 1). In addition to nine design patents, a final utility patent for the pillbox is currently pending.

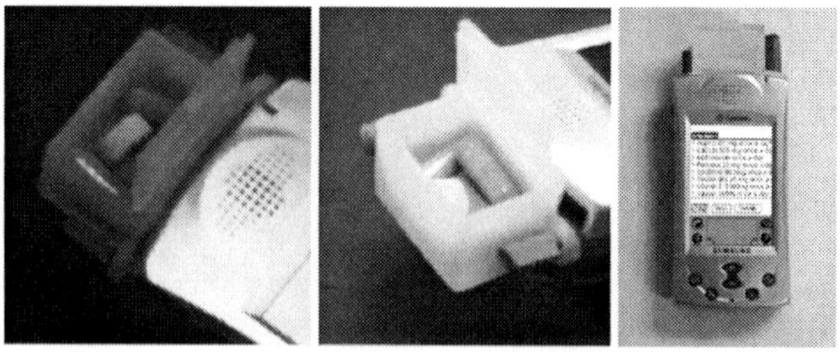

Figure 1. The PDA Pillbox Prototype (patent pending) on the Samsung i300. The PDA pillbox could hold a day's worth of pills, improved access to the stylus, and allowed wireless infrared transfer of information between devices.

1. Improving Medication Adherence Through the Design of the RxReminder™ Software

The most important design principle we focused on was connecting instructions and information to the medication. The most serious drawback of traditional pillboxes is they separate medication from the dosage and consumption instructions (e.g. take with water) and warnings (e.g. not to be taken with grapefruit juice).

To connect the medication and instructions, we began by making the application capable of showing pictures of drugs. The shape, color, and markings of the pills can be clearly seen by the individual. When looking at the details of a particular medication the name, dosage, number of tablets or capsules, and the reason for taking the pills are clearly presented. Contact information for the doctor, pharmacy, and a running pill count are also featured.

We recognize it is possible to program alarms to perform this kind of scheduling. However, it would not provide a picture, a doctor contact, an automatic pill count and many other features possible with the program. Further, RxReminder™ is designed for older adults. All buttons and text are oversized. We use a 14-point font where possible to improve readability. Key screens are presented in Figure 2.

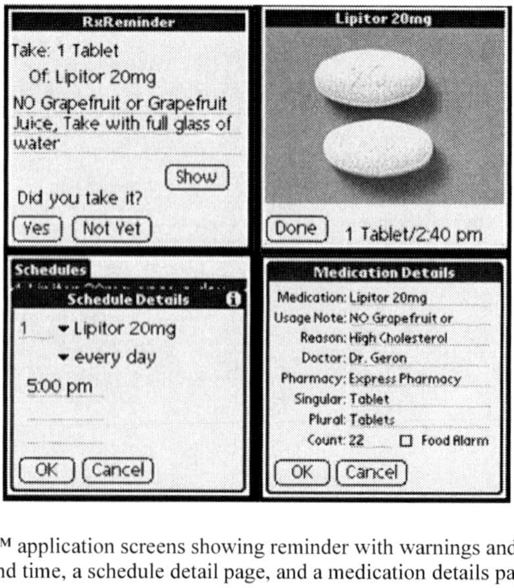

Figure 2. Key RxReminder™ application screens showing reminder with warnings and instructions, a picture with dosage and time, a schedule detail page, and a medication details page

2. The PDA Pillbox

The final step in linking the information in the PDA to the medications was to provide a place to store and carry the medication. We designed a pillbox attachment that would integrate with the PDA and make the stylus more accessible to older users. The PDA pillbox was designed to carry a daily dose of pills. Most people take their medications in the morning as they prepare for the day and at night as they prepare for bed. Mid-day medications are the most challenging. The idea of the PDA pillbox was to provide a way to carry mid-day medications or supplements. The prototype pillboxes are shown in Figure 1.

3. Study Design

Participants. A total of 49 older adults were recruited and 44 (90%) completed the training. Participants ranged in age from 56 to 89 with an average age of 72 years. A majority of the participants were female (65%). All of the older adults were community based.

The group had more experience with technology then the average elder population. Most had used computers for e-mail or the Internet (76%) and about half had used cell phones (53%). Approximately 25% had no exposure to either computers or cell phones. All participants indicated an interest in learning to use a PDA.

Procedures and Measurements. Training procedures and results are documented in *Evaluation of a Curriculum Design and Program to Train Older Adults to Use Personal Digital Assistants* [4]. Participants were asked to bring two prescriptions if they took 2 or more, 1 prescription if it was the only one they took, or 1 supplement if they took no prescribed medications. A physical count of the pills using a pharmacy tray was conducted for the participants.

Following training, the participants carried the PDA's with them for 3 months. The RxReminder™ sounded alarms according to the individual's regimen. At the end of each 30-day period, the participant returned for an interview. The participants completed a PDA usage questionnaire and physical pill count was conducted on the medications being followed.

4. Results

Medication Adherence Results. Based on the number of physical pill counts the average missed pills were 1.04, 2.43, and .05 pills in months 1, 2, and 3 respectively. A T-test for single means was non-significant indicating that these results were not different from zero. Participants commented that they had become increasingly conscientious about taking their pills with the PDA. Although there was considerable variance in the number of pills over or under each month, we found that 24 individuals, 57% of those counted in the third month of the study had perfect adherence and 28 individuals, 67% of those counted in the third month had missed no more then one pill. Eleven of twelve (92%) of those who took mid-day pills used the pillbox.

We want to emphasize that most individuals, especially those on supplements only, even when doctor recommended, were not rigorous in taking their medications prior to joining the study. Participants universally indicated that they had dramatically improved the regularity of taking their medications at the end of the study.

Usage and Rating the Applications User Interface. Individuals were asked what programs they used. RxReminder™ was used by 93% of participants, significantly higher then other applications. This is certainly influenced by the requirements of the study. Each month participants were asked to rank the applications they used on a 5-point scale where 5 was very easy to use and 1 was very difficult to use. RxReminder™ received the highest rating with an average of 4.4. The Date Book application received a score of 4.2. The Address Book received a score of 4.0. This seems to demonstrate that applying design principles and guidelines does result in software that older adults perceived to be easy to use.

Acknowledgements

This research was supported by the National Institute on Aging, grant number 1R43AG19558-01A2 to Creative Action LLC.

I would like to thank Scott Collins, Kyle Allen, M. D. Ronni Sterns, Ph. D. and Martin Murphy, Ph. D. for contributions as this research was developed and completed. I would also like to thank Vincent Antenucci, Anton Yachmenev, Jeanne Mattern, Ph. D., and Debbie Hoskinson who helped in training and data gathering.

References

[1] Czaja, S. J. & Lee, Chin Chin (2001). The Internet and older adults: Design challenges and opportunities. In N. Charness and D. Park (Eds.), *Communication, technology and aging: Opportunities and challenges for the future*. p. 60-78. Springer Publishing Co, Inc: NY, NY.

[2] Fischer, S., Stewart, T.E., Mehta, S., Wax, R., and Lapinsky, S.E. (2003). Handheld computing in medicine. *Journal of the American Medical Informatics Association*. 10(2): 139-49.

[3] ICADI (2003). Proceedings of the International Conference on Aging & Disability (ICADI). Washington D.C., December 4-6.

[4] Sterns, A. A., (In Press). Evaluation of a Curriculum Design and Program to Train Older Adults to Use Personal Digital Assistants. *The Gerontologist*.

Promoting Independence for Older Persons with Disabilities
W.C. Mann and A. Helal (Eds.)
IOS Press, 2006

Author Index